Living Lighter

Your Guide to a Healthier Weight

From Awareness to Behavior to Change

Living Lighter

Your Guide to a Healthier Weight

From Awareness to Behavior to Change

Authored By,

Kavita Goyal, MD

Sandeep Bansal, MD

WINGS PUBLICATION INTERNATIONAL

WE GIVE WINGS TO YOUR DREAM!

Disclaimer

WINGS PUBLICATION INTERNATIONAL
WE GIVE WINGS TO YOUR DREAM!

Registered Office- Wings Publication International
Sharjah Publishing City, Sharjah, United Arab Emirate (UAE)
Website: http://www. wingspublication. com
Email: mybook@wingspublication. com

First Published by **WINGS PUBLICATION INTERNATIONAL 2026**

Title: **LIVING LIGHTER - YOUR GUIDE TO A HEALTHIER WEIGHT**

Price: ₹999 | $14.99

ISBN 978-93-6006-642-0

Authors' Note

Some portions of this book (including certain images and supporting text) were created with the assistance of AI tools. All content was reviewed, curated, and finalized by the authors.

DEDICATION

To our patients - your courage to change inspires us every day.

To our families - thank you for your love, patience, and unwavering support.

And to anyone ready to take the first step - this is for you. May this book remind you that transformation begins the moment you decide to try. Every choice, no matter how small, is a victory. Every step forward is a testament to your strength. Believe in your ability to grow, and know that you already hold the power to create the life and health you deserve.

Kavita Goyal, MD

Sandeep Bansal, MD

ABOUT THE AUTHORS

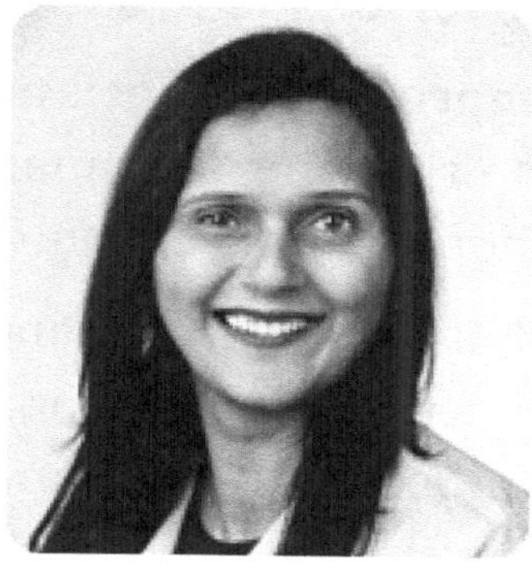

Kavita Goyal, MD

Dr. Kavita Goyal is a double board-certified physician in Internal Medicine and Obesity Medicine. Known for her compassionate, patient-centered approach, she has guided countless individuals toward reclaiming their health by addressing the root causes of weight struggles and chronic disease.

Her expertise lies in combining evidence-based obesity medicine with practical, sustainable strategies. **She has developed innovative group visit models, patient education modules, and community-based programs that empower patients to take charge of their health.** Dr. Goyal's leadership in medical weight management integrates advanced clinical knowledge with practical lifestyle interventions that work in the real world.

In addition to her clinical work, Dr. Goyal actively contributes to the field by teaching, mentoring, and creating educational materials for physicians and patients. She is passionate about making complex medical ideas clear and practical, giving people the knowledge and tools they need for long-term success.

She believes weight management is not about perfection but about progress - showing that small, consistent steps can lead to meaningful, lasting change.

Outside the work Dr. Goyal loves spending time learning Indian classical dance and meditation. Sitting in silence is a perfect way to take a break from day-to-day stress and strongly advises everyone to make it a daily practice.

ABOUT THE AUTHORS

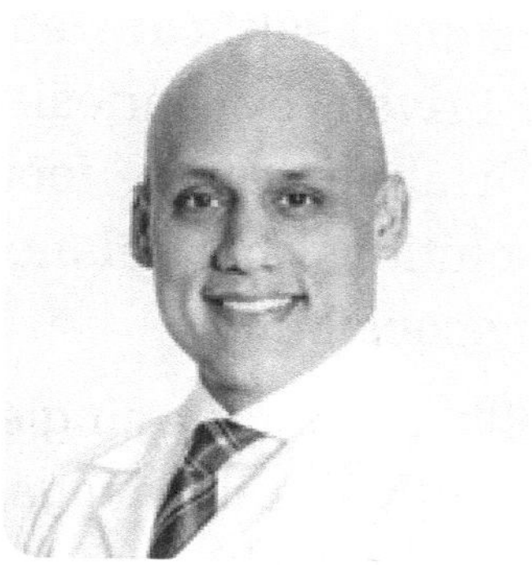

Sandeep Bansal, MD

Dr. Sandeep Bansal is an author, entrepreneur, innovator and physician leader dedicated to improving patient outcomes through innovation, empathy, and personalized care. He created **The ABC Technique - a practical framework built around Awareness, Behavior, and Change - designed to help individuals achieve lasting health transformations.**

Throughout his career, Dr. Bansal has combined clinical expertise with healthcare innovation. He leads several organizations that together deliver comprehensive services ranging from outpatient and inpatient care to advanced clinical research, including the use of genomics and robotics for early disease detection and treatment.

A specialist in Internal Medicine, Critical Care, Pulmonary Disease and Sleep Disorders, Dr. Bansal has developed systems of care that are both high-tech and high-touch, ensuring that advanced treatments remain compassionate and meaningful for patients.

Beyond clinical practice, his expertise includes **organizational design, healthcare strategy, and start-up development.** Driven by curiosity and a passion for reimagining healthcare, he focuses on creating patient-centered solutions that balance innovation with compassion and responsibility.

At the heart of all his work is a single guiding principle: **to empower people with the knowledge, tools, and support to take control of their health and unlock their fullest potential.**

Outside of work, Dr. Bansal enjoys meditation, music, hiking in nature, traveling to new places, and exploring different cultures. These practices not only provide restoration and perspective but also deepen his understanding of the human experience.

Together, Dr. Goyal and Dr. Bansal bring more than four decades of combined experience to Living Lighter. Blending clinical expertise, behavioral insight, and a whole-person approach, they have created a guide that is rooted in science, infused with compassion, and designed to empower readers to transform their health, one meaningful step at a time.

ABOUT THE BOOK

Living Lighter: Your Guide to a Healthier Weight is more than a weight loss book - it's a physician-developed roadmap for sustainable transformation. Rooted in clinical expertise and behavioral science, it offers readers the tools to take charge of their health, not just by shedding pounds but by reshaping their mindset and habits for lasting well-being.

Organized into three sections - **what, why, and how** - this guide begins by explaining the science behind obesity and its connection to inflammation and chronic illness. It then examines the reasons behind weight struggles, focusing on behavioral patterns that keep us stuck. The practical third section introduces strategies for lasting success, emphasizing four pillars: diet, exercise, behavior, and medication.

At its core is the **ABC Technique - Awareness, Behavior, Change** - A straightforward method for recognizing habits, making purposeful adjustments, and achieving sustainable results. Each section concludes with interactive ABC Technique exercises, empowering readers to put concepts into action. Whether your goals are to lose weight, manage stress, enhance sleep, or overcome emotional and substance-driven habits, this technique offers clear steps for lasting transformation.

Inside, readers will discover:

- The biological, emotional, and environmental factors behind weight gain
- Tools to overcome cravings, food addiction, and emotional eating
- Habits that support lasting changes in nutrition, movement, and mindset
- Guidance on weight loss medications and surgical options
- Reflective prompts to deepen self-awareness and motivation

Living Lighter is a practical guide for anyone ready to shed both physical and emotional weight - and step into lasting transformation.

PREFACE

We wrote ***Living Lighter*** because we have witnessed the struggle firsthand - not only as physicians, but as human beings committed to health, healing, and human consciousness.

For years, we've watched patients carry more than just physical weight. The burden often includes guilt, confusion, frustration, and a quiet sense of failure. And yet, every person's story is layered with effort, resilience, and the hope for change.

This book is our response to those stories.

The human brain contains approximately 82 billion neurons, making it the most intricate and advanced organ among all living beings. It is an incredible tool - capable of creativity, compassion, and problem-solving at a level unmatched in the natural world. Yet, like any powerful tool, it can only serve us well if we learn how to handle it. A knife in the wrong grip becomes dangerous, but in skilled hands it becomes a remarkable gift. If neglected or conditioned in unconstructive ways, the same mind can trap us in cycles of stress, poor habits, and unhealthy behaviors. In the same way, our minds, if used with awareness and care, can help us lead joyful, fulfilling lives.

If we stop and think, many of us see the same pattern in our lives. Even with all the new tools, social media apps, and health advice around us, our daily lives still feel stressful and overwhelming. We set goals to eat better, exercise more, or get enough sleep - but often fall back into old habits. It can feel frustrating, like we're standing in our own way.

From childhood, our brains are hardwired by family, culture, and experiences. Over time, these patterns become automatic - how we eat, how we handle stress, even how we respond to emotions. The good news is that these habits are not permanent. They can be noticed, understood, and slowly reshaped.

That's what this book is here to help you do. We'll guide you to recognize the patterns that may be holding you back and show you simple, practical steps to change them. Our goal is not to overwhelm you with medical terms, but to give you clear tools and encouragement. When you understand how your mind and body work, it becomes easier to make changes that last.

To make the journey clear, the book is organized into three sections - ***what, why, and how.*** First, we explain the science behind obesity and how it connects to inflammation and long-term health conditions. Next, we explore the reasons so many people struggle with weight, focusing on the behaviors and habits that keep us stuck. Finally, in the practical third section, we introduce strategies for lasting success, built around four key pillars: diet, exercise, behavior, and medication.

Living Lighter isn't a quick-fix program or a rigid prescription. It's a guide rooted in science, compassion, and the belief that lasting transformation comes from understanding — not shame. At the heart of it all is the **ABC Technique - Awareness, Behavior, and Change.**

The **ABC framework** is simple but powerful. It begins with **Awareness**: recognizing your patterns, your triggers, and the choices that shape your health. From there, it moves into **Behavior:** taking intentional, practical steps that align with your goals. Finally, it guides you to **Change**: building momentum with real-life tools such as:

- **Mindful eating and nutrition guidance** - slowing down to notice hunger cues, enjoying food without guilt, and learning how to overcome weight-loss plateaus. This section also helps you understand your body's nutritional needs, with clear explanations of macronutrients and micronutrients, healthy options for carbs, fats, proteins, and fiber, as well as insights into different diet approaches and alternative, easier ways to lose weight.
- **Practical movement strategies** - from simple seated exercises to higher-intensity workouts, making physical activity realistic, sustainable, and adaptable to your lifestyle - even when time feels limited.
- **Stress-management tools** - such as mindful breathing, journaling, and meditation, to help you handle stress and break the cycle that links emotions to unhealthy habits.

- **Better sleep routines** - with practical tips to restore your body's natural rhythms, improve energy, and support long-term health.
- **Medication and treatment options** - explained in clear, accessible language, so you can make informed decisions about medical support when appropriate.

Together, these tools lead to sustainable results and a lighter, healthier life - not just physically, but mentally and emotionally as well.

What makes the ABC Technique unique is its flexibility. While deeply grounded in the science of obesity and weight management, it applies to nearly every area of life where transformation is needed - from managing stress and improving sleep to reshaping habits and even letting go of unhealthy dependencies.

Throughout this book, each section closes with a guided ABC application, so you can turn insight into action and see measurable progress in your own journey.

We don't just want you to lose weight - we want you to feel lighter in every sense of the word.

Thank you for allowing us to be part of your journey. May these pages help you take your first - and next - steps with clarity, courage, and hope.

Kavita Goyal, MD

Sandeep Bansal, MD

INDEX

Chapter : 1

Introduction

"The journey of a thousand miles begins with a single step."

-Lao Tzu

A CLINICAL TURNING POINT

A vivid memory like this never fades.

In 2016, a 46-year-old man's life nearly ended in an instant. Alone in his trailer, he was struck by sudden, crushing chest pain and gasping breath. Terrified but determined, he reached for the phone and called 911.

When emergency responders arrived, they quickly realized the challenge. At nearly 550 pounds, he couldn't fit through the narrow doorway. Time was critical, and the team had to act fast. In a moment of extraordinary teamwork and urgency, they cut through the side of his trailer to get him out safely and rush him to the hospital.

Upon arrival at the emergency department, the patient's oxygen levels were critically low, and he continued to struggle for breath, though his chest pain had subsided. He was immediately placed on supplemental oxygen. Due to the severity of his respiratory distress, he was transferred to intensive care unit (ICU) under my care for closer monitoring and advanced care.

The patient's size presented significant challenges. He could barely fit into the hospital bed, and standard equipment was often inadequate. Despite initial stabilization, his oxygen levels began to drop again within an hour of arrival, and he showed signs of a heart attack. A rapid response team was activated. We provided critical interventions he needed. Over the next few days, his condition steadily improved. He was weaned off the ventilator and eventually made a full recovery from this life-threatening episode.

This challenging case highlights the medical complexities of caring for patients with extreme obesity.

A few days later, the patient returned to our clinic for follow-up. Seated in a wheelchair with a downcast head, he appeared visibly sad and still weighed over 500 pounds.

The patient's medical chart listed several conditions related to weight gain. Following the completion of a routine medical examination, we engaged in a detailed discussion regarding the circumstances that led to this significant increase in weight. I recall distinctly that he looked me in the eyes and remarked, "Doc, I have always found comfort in food. I ate when I was happy. I ate when I was sad. I just didn't know any other way to cope. Now, I can barely walk and am bound to this chair."

We took decisive steps to support him in his future journey. We began by discussing his diet. Given his complete reliance on others for daily needs, his family would provide better food options within his reach. Weight loss medications were not covered by the insurance, but his recent life-threatening illness made him determined to make changes in his lifestyle.

This experience highlighted the need for us to take more proactive measures in our practices. We looked at several resources and have since made significant advances toward helping our patients achieve their weight loss goals. The insights we share in this book are grounded not only in research and clinical expertise but also in our extensive experience working with hundreds of patients over the past several years. We are confident that the knowledge we have gained will make a meaningful impact.

As physicians, we face many challenges, especially providing comprehensive care within the allotted time frame. For us, experience in weight management works as a tool to provide the best care to our patients, giving them everything they need to transition from a condition to a conscious and healthy life. There are many aspects to this journey, most importantly, working on the hardwiring of your mind. It includes breaking difficult habits and mental conditioning that keep us trapped in cycles and patterns of life that are crucial to break to live a truly authentic life.

This book is divided into three parts: ***what, why, and how.*** In the first part, we discuss what obesity is and how it has become a national epidemic. We will review basic facts about this disease. The second part, why, is focused on the importance of understanding the impacts of unhealthy weight gain on our bodies. The final part, how, is most crucial and most extensive in this book, where we talk about ways to work on losing weight and gaining health. Four pillars of weight management, including diet, exercise, behavior, and medications, are discussed individually.

In each section of the book, we will provide you with a practical, evidence-informed guide using the **ABC**

Technique - a 3-step method that empowers readers to move from insight to action to lasting transformation. This book bridges medicine, mindset, and everyday choices to help you become Aware your patterns, shift your Behaviors, and embrace sustainable Change.

The ABC technique:

A - Awareness → B - Behavior → C - Change

A - Awareness:

"See it clearly. Before you change what you do, understand why you do it. "

B - Behavior: Build New Habits

"Start with small steps, stay consistent, and stack habits that matter."

C - Change: Sustain and Transform

"Real transformation happens when your choices reflect who you believe yourself to be, not just your willpower."

Under each step, you are given reflection prompts for you to make your own journal entries to help you with this journey. These prompts are not all inclusive. We encourage you to be creative and add your own thoughts.

To get the most out of this book, please refer to the index to identify your current struggle that you are working on. Choose your topic and focus on that. The journey is not limited to losing weight. It is about reinventing yourself by breaking free from all the hardwiring and conditioning that do not align with your soul. It is about welcoming who you are meant to be while serving a purpose in this divine life.

Back to our patient: with courage, determination, and support of his family, he embraced profound lifestyle changes. In just six months, he shed 100 pounds - a milestone that opened the door to bariatric surgery. Three years later, his journey has taken him from 550 pounds to 250. Today, he is not only lighter in body but freer in spirit. Unrestricted from many of the chronic ailments that once held him back, he now radiates happiness, resilience, and a renewed sense of purpose. His story is proof that transformation is possible, and that every step forward - no matter how difficult - can lead to a brighter, healthier life.

OBESITY EPIDEMIC IN THE UNITED STATES

The definition of epidemic is a rapid outspread of a disease to a large number of hosts in a given population within a short period of time. For example, the COVID-19 epidemic, which we experienced a few years ago.

The following is the graph of the obesity epidemic in the US:

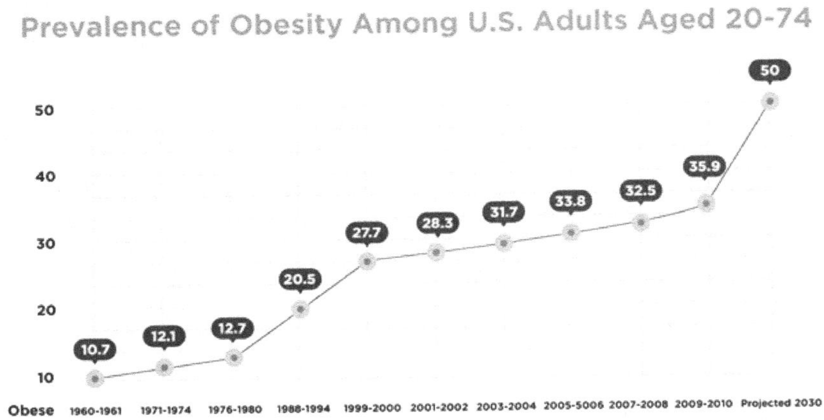

Derived from NHANES data (http://www.cdc.gov/nchs/data/hestat/obesity_adult_09_10/obesity_adult_09_10.html#table1)

If we pay attention to this obesity graph, we can see that the rate of obesity really started rising after the 1990s. Prior to that, the rate was around 10%. By 2040, we are expecting the number to rise to 50%. Every other person in America is going to be dealing with unhealthy weight gain.

This is an extremely worrying statistic. America was ranked number 10 by World Obesity Data, with a 41.5% obesity rate in 2023. It has risen sharply since the 1990s, from almost 15% to 41%.

If we really think about it, we have better technology, better equipment, better diet options, and better exercise plans loaded in our smartphones. There is more money spent on healthcare. Despite all this, obesity has been increasing at an alarming rate since 1990. Does this mean that we did something fundamentally wrong?

Remember, this is not just a hypothetical graph. There is a person behind each of these numbers and a whole family behind that person. It does not matter where you are in this health journey, whether aiming to lose weight or enhance fitness, it is essential to be aware of the severity of this epidemic in our country.

Regardless of your profession, you can contribute by providing support to your loved ones, caring for yourself, and helping those around you.

DID WE GET IT ALL WRONG?

Prior to the 1990s, sugar was advertised as an energy source. Refer to this picture taken for a sugar advertisement during the 1970s.

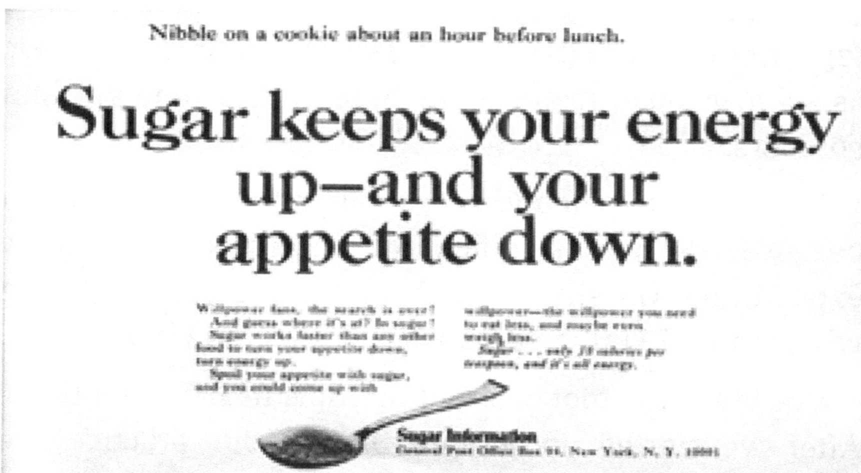
Nibble on a cookie about an hour before lunch.
Sugar keeps your energy up—and your appetite down.
Sugar Information

Sugar was considered a healthy energy source that could help cut down appetite. There was so much emphasis on cutting down the fat that the big elephant in the room, wrapped in a small sugar candy wrapper, got completely ignored. Now we are facing the outcomes. The obesity epidemic has increased from 10% to almost 40% now.

Not enough emphasis was placed on cutting down sugar intake. The easy availability of unhealthy foods, advancements in technology, sitting for long hours, a busy and stressful lifestyle, limited home cooking and no meal prep have ultimately led us to this epidemic.

If you really pay attention, our section for packaged foods in the grocery store is getting bigger, whereas the fresh foods section keeps on shrinking in size. Organic and fresh foods are becoming too expensive for average Americans.

On average, an American sits for eight hours a day. A rapid rise in technology has increased sedentary behavior, as more people spend more time sitting indoors than outdoors.

The obesity epidemic keeps gaining a lot of attention because it has significantly increased healthcare expenditure. Obesity costs the US healthcare system a whopping $173 billion a year, as per CDC data in 2023.

Obesity is the root cause of multiple health conditions. After we started addressing BMI in our practice, we understood that we were finally treating the root of the disease and not just the symptoms. Many patients stopped using their CPAP machines. Their diabetes, hypertension, fatty liver disease, and most importantly, their self-esteem improved significantly.

There is certainly more awareness of this diseased state. The government is trying its best to fight this condition. Obesity Medical Association is working hard to bring this awareness among physicians and provide them with tools to incorporate obesity treatment in their routine medical practice.

We achieve greater success when we learn from our past mistakes. We now clearly understand sugar's harmful impact on our health. There is a whole chapter dedicated to sugar and its effects on the body in this book. We have recommended a daily dose for sugar intake, but that doesn't work for a mind that is addicted to sugar. We need to watch our sugar intake personally and encourage all our friends and loved ones to adopt this habit as part of their lifestyle. A dinner table discussion can raise awareness about sugar intake. Talking about it to our kids can go a long way towards achieving a positive change.

Remember, family is the smallest unit of a nation.

A healthy family contributes to a healthy nation.

LEARN FROM OTHERS

Brian (name changed) is a 45-year-old man. He is the owner of a reputable restaurant in town. He works tirelessly day and night to keep up with the business requirements. His documented BMI is close to 40. Being 6'7" inches tall, He really made me feel short, though I am 5'7". Being the owner and working in a restaurant, Brian would have no time to have breakfast or lunch. He would have one hearty meal at the end of his day; whatever was available in his bakery. While he was providing healthy salads, chicken, and egg sandwiches to everyone in the cafeteria, he barely had any time for himself. His dinner would consist of lots of bread, potatoes, spaghetti, pizza, and chicken, loads of carbohydrates. He admitted to eating a large meal at the end of his day, which was close to 3000 calories.

At his first visit, we identified a key trigger behind his weight gain. Instead of asking him to change everything at once, we focused on making just one small change at a time. His cafeteria staff helped by providing healthy, portion-controlled meals for breakfast and lunch, such as an egg sandwich in the morning and a small plate of chicken salad in the afternoon.

At dinner, the goal was straightforward: cut back on bread and carbohydrates by half. He followed this plan consistently and often went beyond what was recommended. Over time, his nighttime carbohydrate intake dropped significantly, allowing steady and sustainable progress rather than extreme restriction.

Weight-loss medications were also started and played an important role by helping control his appetite and support these lifestyle changes. Over the next 12 months, he lost nearly 80 pounds.

As the weight came off, his health improved significantly. He needed much less support from his CPAP machine, and he was able to stop his blood pressure medications altogether.

This experience shows how small, focused behavior changes, when paired with the right medical support, can lead to lasting, life-changing results.

He is still on his journey, plateauing at times and losing weight off and on. Losing 80 pounds with lifestyle interventions and medications is absolutely remarkable. He had access to healthy food options in his cafeteria and began using them effectively, achieving his goals as a result.

The skipping of breakfast and lunch, combined with the consumption of one large dinner, is commonly observed among my patients dealing with weight issues. Highly refined sugars and carbohydrates are typically included in this dinner, along with prolonged periods of sitting (8-10 hours) due to job requirements and busy lifestyles. Significant stress and emotional eating are also frequently experienced. People often choose comfort foods that are rich in refined carbs and high degree of fat because they are easy, inexpensive, and palatable. It takes conscious efforts to identify and break the patterns of unhealthy eating habits.

At his first visit, we identified a key trigger behind his weight gain. Instead of asking him to change everything at once, we focused on making just one small change at a time. His cafeteria staff helped by providing healthy, portion-controlled meals for breakfast and lunch, such as an egg sandwich in the morning and a small plate of chicken salad in the afternoon.

At dinner, the goal was straightforward: cut back

on bread and carbohydrates by half. He followed this plan consistently and often went beyond what was recommended. Over time, his nighttime carbohydrate intake dropped significantly, allowing steady and sustainable progress rather than extreme restriction.

Weight-loss medications were also started and played an important role by helping control his appetite and support these lifestyle changes. Over the next 12 months, he lost nearly 80 pounds.

As the weight came off, his health improved significantly. He needed much less support from his CPAP machine, and he was able to stop his blood pressure medications altogether.

This experience shows how small, focused behavior changes, when paired with the right medical support, can lead to lasting, life-changing results.

Take a moment to identify relevant factors from the case example provided. Bringing this to your awareness can help you build new behaviors and finally making a lasting change.

Chapter : 2

Understanding Obesity

*"If you can't explain it simply,
you don't understand it well enough"*

-Albert Einstein

WHAT THE NUMBERS DON'T TELL YOU

Let us understand what obesity exactly is and what is the science behind it. In this chapter, we will also discuss obesity related conditions, mainly it being a high inflammatory state.

What is Obesity?

Obesity is a chronic condition characterized by an excessive accumulation of body fat that poses a significant risk to health.

To understand this disease, we need to get familiar with a few medical terms that are usually used, not only in medical offices but also in routine conversations alike. You may have heard of BMI (body mass index), BMR (basal metabolic rate), lean mass, insulin resistance, etc. Your doctor will often use these words while discussing this condition with you.

2.1: 3 THINGS YOU MUST KNOW ABOUT YOUR BODY

1. **BMI:** BMI measures your weight relative to your height, calculated as weight divided by height squared. The result falls into three classes of obesity. Class 1 BMI ranges between 30-35, class 2 is 35-40, and class 3 is BMI above 40. A BMI between 25 to 30 is classified as

overweight per medical standards.

Normal Weight 18.5- 24.9	Overweight 25.0- 29.9	Class I Obesity 30.0- 34.9	Class II Obesity 35.0- 39.9	Class III Obesity > 40

BMI category varies from country to country. For example, in Asian countries, any BMI above 27 is considered high.

2. BODY COMPOSITION: The second thing that you must know about your body is body composition. See the picture below:

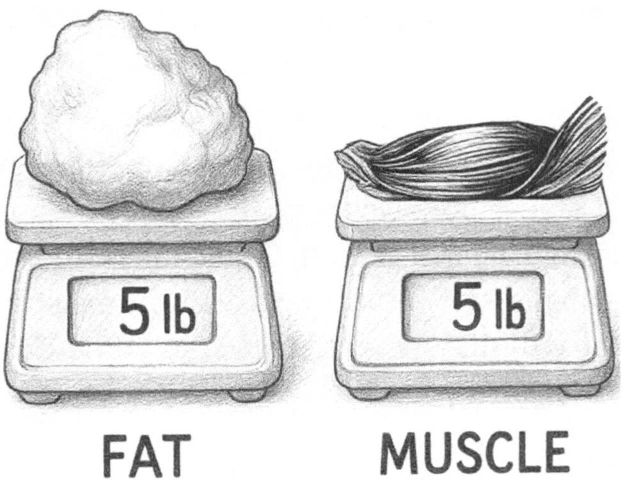

Two people could have the same height, weight, and BMI but totally different body compositions. As you can see in this picture, these two weights are exactly the same, but one is all fat and the other is pure muscle. BMI by itself does not give a complete picture until we study the body composition as well. There are many ways to know your body composition, i.e., knowing your fat mass, lean mass, muscle mass, body water, BMR, etc. A body composition scale is available on the market that can give you a body composition. Many physicians use body composition scales in their practices, so you may consult your doctor for additional details.

The biggest advantage of doing body composition during your weight loss journey is that when you lose weight, you can make sure you are not losing your lean mass. If someone is losing weight by starvation or not having enough protein, we see a decrease in lean mass along with the weight loss. That is an unhealthy way of losing weight. Here is an example of body composition from our practice when a patient lost significant weight, and we repeated body composition to check the lean mass and total body water.

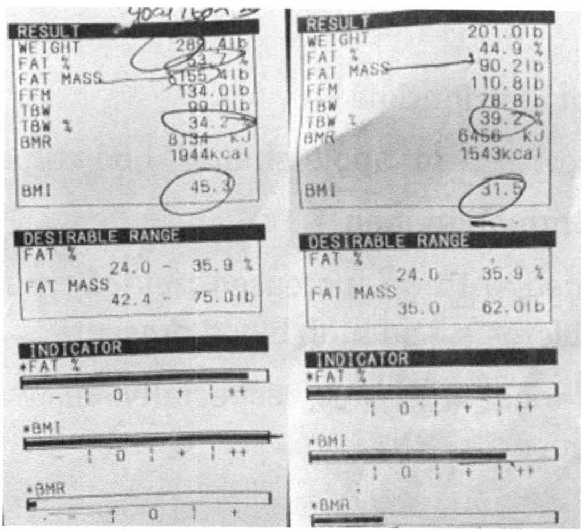

3. BODY TYPE: Body type depends on fat distribution.

If the fat distribution is more around the waist, it is called android. It is more common in men. If the fat distribution is more around the hip area, it is called gynoid (also known as gluteal femoral), which is more common in women.

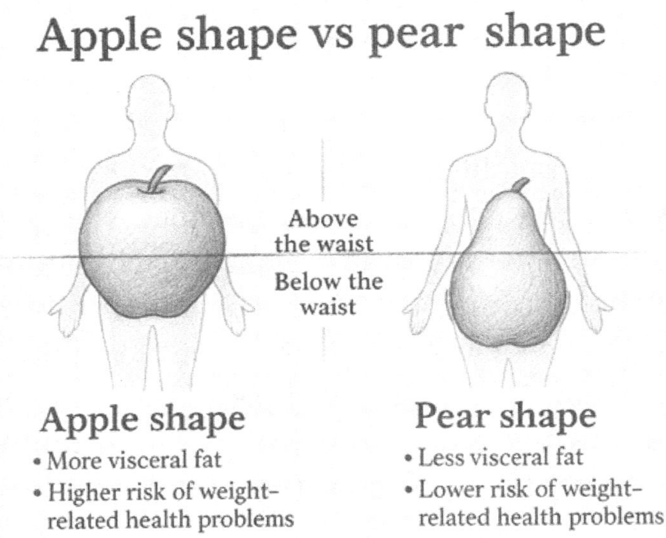

Android fat distribution:

- Also known as an "apple-shaped" body type
- More common in men
- Associated with an increased risk of type 2 diabetes, atherosclerosis, and high blood pressure
- Can change with age, especially in women after menopause

Gynoid fat distribution (Gluteal femoral):

- Also known as a "pear-shaped" body type
- In women, this distribution pattern is primarily determined by estrogen levels

Why is it important?

In a gynoid type of body, fat is found more around the hip area. It is not associated with increased cardiovascular conditions. When the waist-to-hip ratio is high and there is more fat around the waist, it is associated with increased cardiovascular conditions and called an android-type body.

Women have a high tendency to store fat around the hips and thighs, called gynoid. This is primarily genetic. Men tend to have higher abdominal fat, called an android-type body. Hip fat is generally hard to lose.

2.2 OBESITY RELATED COMORBIDITIES

1. Fatty liver disease

This disease state is also called MASLD (Metabolic Dysfunction-Associated Steatotic Liver Disease). For the sake of simplicity and better understanding, we'll use the term Fatty liver disease in this section.

Angela (name changed), a 22-year-old girl, saw us for weight management, hepatic steatosis, and fatty liver disease. This is a relatively frequent occurrence, as patients with liver disease are routinely encountered in our clinical practice. However, her age was something that really caught our attention. Developing a liver condition at such an early age was quite surprising.

Angela was found to have an enlarged liver incidentally on an ultrasound. She had earlier complained of abdominal pain. Hence, the ultrasound was performed to rule out kidney stones. Her liver was not only enlarged but also appeared hardened on the ultrasound. She ended up having a biopsy that revealed stage 3 liver disease. Her weight and height placed her in the class 3 category of BMI above 40. This was an eye-opener for Angela. Thus, she actively sought help for weight management and liver disease. The liver specialist (hepatologist) recommended that losing weight was the only option for her to stop her liver disease from progressing.

When we talked, she revealed that she had been raised on a diet containing lots of sweet beverages, sugary doughnuts, and fried foods since the age of 5 (ever since she remembered). Her food list was pretty much the same all her life, on an extensive diet recall. She was raised by a single father who kept busy doing two jobs. Now, at the age of 23, she was ready to make the necessary changes to her diet.

Learning from her past eating habits, Angela seemed willing to do better. We sat down and came up with a strong plan with the help of a nutritionist. She was also started on an exercise plan, along with some medications. Angela is still on her journey, but her diet has changed drastically. Not surprisingly, her liver enzymes are in the normal range. Our primary goal is to help her prevent the progression of this disease.

Let us talk about what fatty liver disease is and how it is associated with unhealthy weight gain.

As the name suggests, the disease is a condition in when fat starts depositing inside liver cells. Around 80% of patients with a BMI above 40 invariably suffer from this condition.

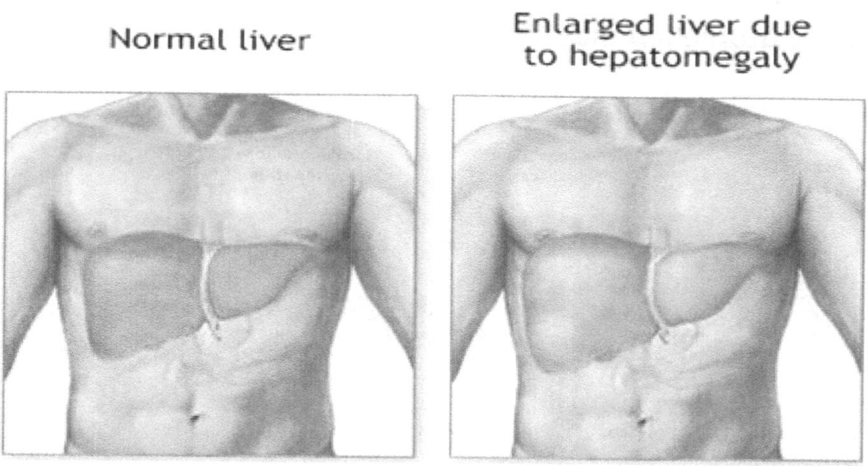

The liver is a soft organ with smooth margins, located on the right upper side of the abdomen. The main function of the liver is to work as a warrior in the body. The liver works as a detoxifying agent if the body is attacked with toxins. It also works as a storage unit for extra calories, carbs, and fats. Whenever we consume food, it is not used as an energy source immediately. It gets stored in the liver in the form of glycogen and fat inside the cells.

As you can see in the first picture, a healthy liver is comprised of well-organized cells. It does not have too many fat cells when observed under a microscope. As fat gets deposited inside the cells, the body develops a condition called fatty liver disease. The liver also starts getting enlarged in the process.

If you do not follow a healthy diet and continue consuming unhealthy, processed, and high amounts of fats and carbohydrates in the diet without working out, all the extra calories keep getting deposited in the liver. As shown in the picture below, fat gets deposited in the form of fat droplets inside the liver cells.

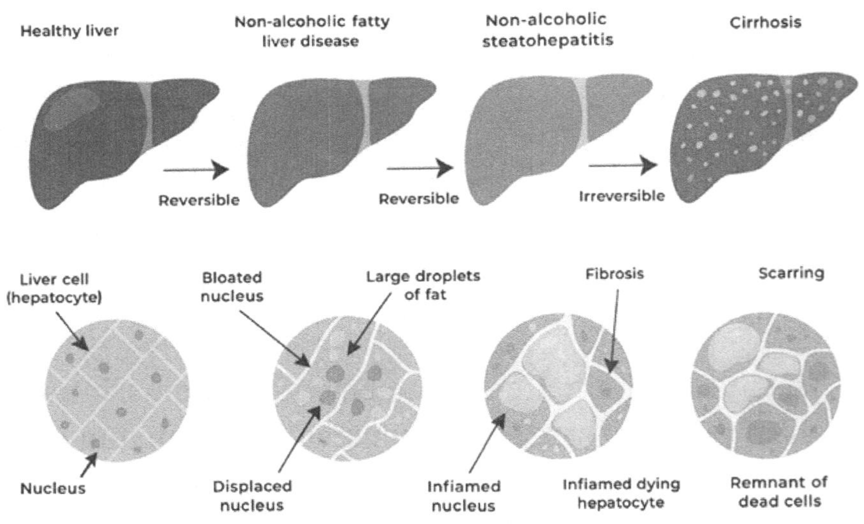

You can see how the liver goes through some structural changes at a microscopic level, leading to inflammation, fibrosis, and color change. The liver starts getting harder, which leads to a condition called hepatic steatosis. It is also associated with inflammation and fibrosis in the cell.

Finally, if we do not start working on our diet and continue gaining weight in unhealthy ways, we get intense scarring with remnants of dead cells in the liver. This releases a lot of liver enzymes into the bloodstream. This is where patients develop a condition called hepatic cirrhosis that is almost irreversible. Liver margins become irregular, and the liver turns from a soft, smooth organ into a harder organ with lots of scarring.

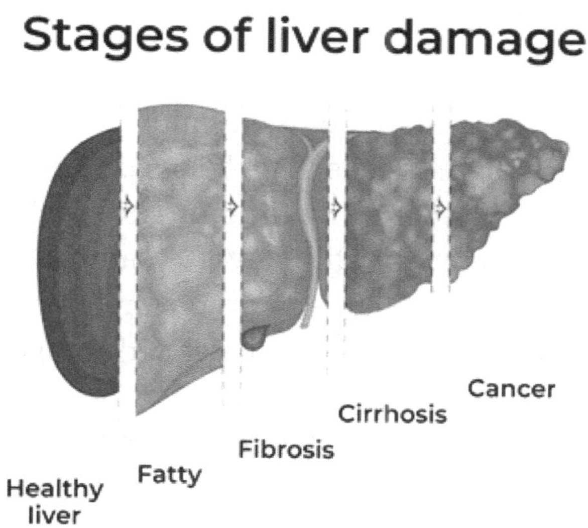

Source: https://medicine.washu.edu/news/study-reveals-links-between-fatty-liver-disease-liver-cancer

The most important aspect of this disease condition is that fatty liver disease and hepatic steatosis are reversible. It can be controlled with lifestyle modifications, interventions, and weight. However, if the condition further regresses into cirrhosis, it becomes **an irreversible liver disease.**

HOW TO FIND IF YOU HAVE MSALD:

If you are dealing with high BMI or unhealthy weight gain, you should get your liver enzymes checked. You can always ask your provider to run a blood test. This disease can be diagnosed with an ultrasound. Individuals with weight concerns and a BMI over 40 should consider this option.

WHAT CAN YOU ABOUT IT:

If you are diagnosed with this condition, you must immediately consult a dietitian and work towards a healthier diet plan. Please find below some foods that will help alleviate this condition. The basic concept and key in this journey still stay the same, i.e., limiting and cutting down on refined carbohydrates and sugary beverages and incorporating a balanced intake of fruits, vegetables, whole grains, lean proteins, and healthy fats. The Mediterranean diet is also considered healthy for the liver. Please refer to the section 4.8 for details.

Please scan the QR code for liver friendly diet and healthy recipes from American liver foundation.

FOODS THAT HELP CLEANSING THE LIVER

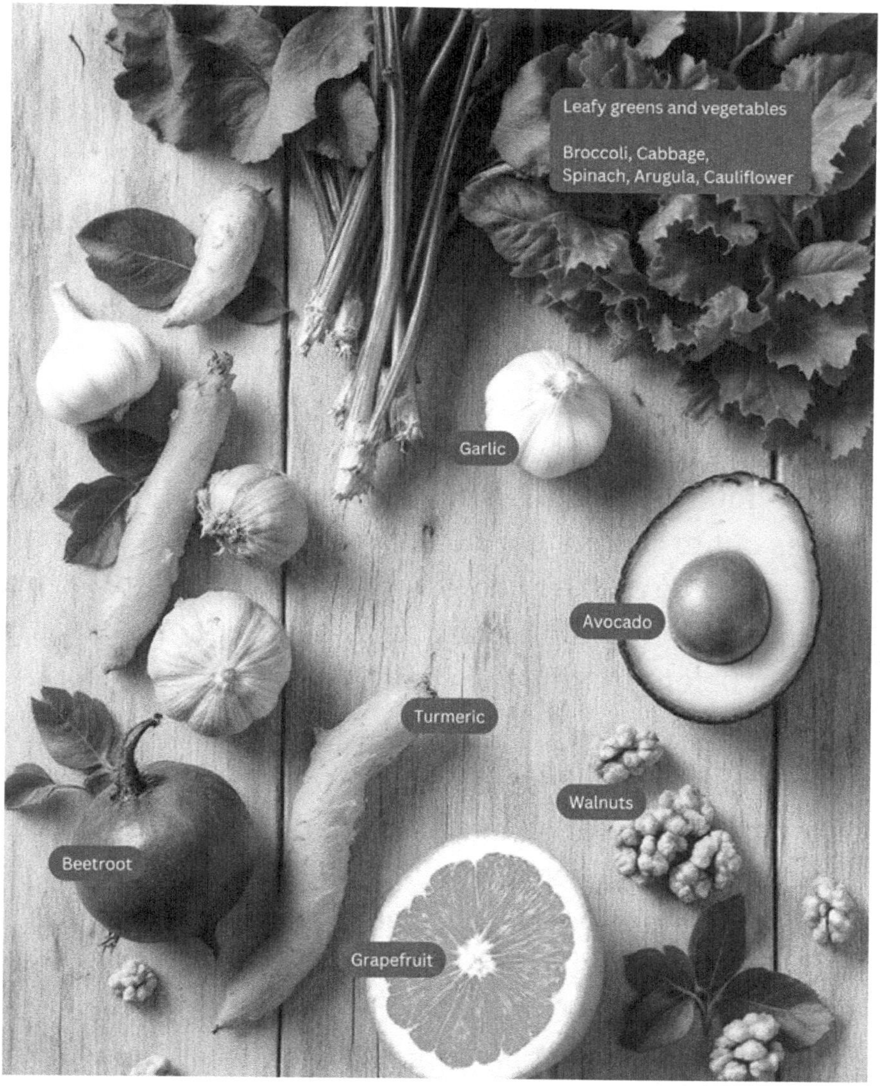
Leafy greens and vegetables
Broccoli, Cabbage,
Spinach, Arugula, Cauliflower
Garlic
Avocado
Turmeric
Walnuts
Beetroot
Grapefruit

Here we are talking mainly about non-alcoholic fatty liver disease. Liver disease can also be caused due to medications or alcohol. See the section 4.7 on impact of alcohol on obesity.

About 85% of people with a body mass index (BMI) of 40 or higher have non-alcoholic fatty liver disease (NAFLD).

2. INSULIN RESISTANCE

Do you know how much sugar is in your bloodstream? Pause briefly and consider your average daily sugar intake. Typical responses we get, often range from 50 to 100 grams; however, the actual amount of sugar present in the entire bloodstream is approximately one teaspoon, equivalent to 5 milligrams. On average, in a human being who is not diabetic, the blood sugar level varies between 80-100 mg/dL, and the human body has 5 L of blood. It comes out to **5 gram per 5 Liter of blood.** It's a very small amount – like a tiny pinch of sugar in a big bottle of water. You probably wouldn't even taste it. Just remember this number before reading the next statistic.

So, what happens to all this extra sugar that we consume in our bodies? It raises blood sugar to cause diabetes or is stored in the body. The liver stores this extra sugar in the form of fat and glycogen (carbohydrate storage form). If you consume such sugar-rich foods frequently, eventually this results in **fatty liver disease (FLD).** If you have a diagnosis of fatty liver disease or liver cirrhosis, you can directly jump to the chapter on FLD and get to know your liver in more detail. In that chapter, I have also shared tips on how to prevent the progression of this diseased state.

Sugar is used as an immediate energy source by our brain, muscles, and various metabolic functions of our body, but the rest of the unconsumed sugar gets stored in the form of fat within the liver, under the skin, or around internal organs.

Let us now understand what sugar does to our bodies.

Excess sugar consumption increases blood sugar levels, which can lead to insulin resistance. This means your body organs specifically muscles do not respond well to insulin, prompting the pancreas to produce even more. Over time, this chronic overwork can contribute to the development of type 2 diabetes. Additionally, this excess sugar is converted and stored as fat in the liver, contributing to fatty liver disease.

Insulin is a vital hormone that works more like a doorkeeper for the sugar gates in our cells (refer to the picture below).

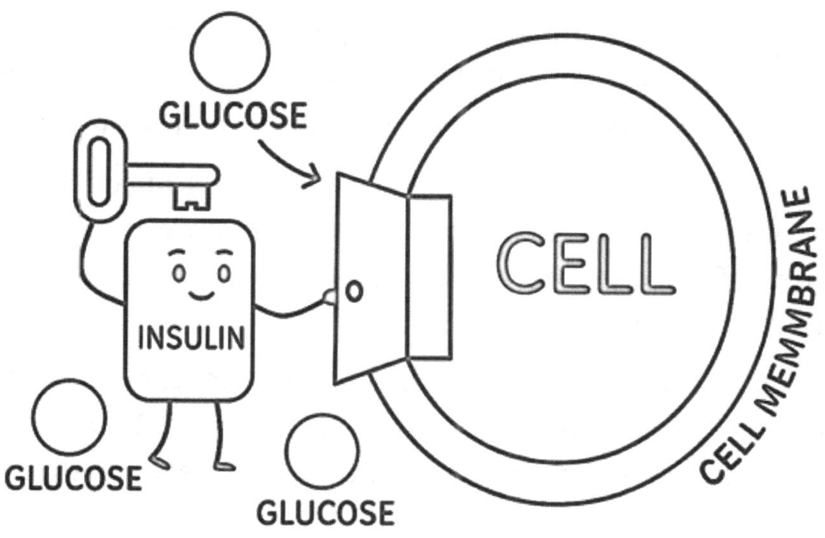

Imagine each of your body's cells as a room, with a door that allows sugar (glucose) to enter and provide energy. **Insulin acts as the doorkeeper**—it unlocks the door so sugar can move from your bloodstream into the cell. This is how your body normally keeps blood sugar levels under control.

When we eat too many refined carbs or sugary foods, the amount of sugar in the blood rises quickly. Suddenly, there's a crowd at the "door" waiting to get in. To handle the traffic, the body creates more doors and calls in more doorkeepers—meaning insulin levels rise. But over time, the cells stop responding as well to insulin's signal. This is called **insulin resistance.**

Think of it this way: if one person can pass through one door, then eating large amounts of sugar is like sending a crowd of people all at once. The doorkeeper (insulin) struggles to manage the flow, especially when the "room" (your cell) is already full. The sugar can't get inside, but the insulin levels keep climbing, and blood sugar level rises.

Even if you're not eating huge amounts of food, high insulin locks the doors and prevents energy from being used efficiently. The result? Fatigue, weight gain, and a state of chronic inflammation.

Over time, insulin resistance can set the stage for serious health problems—including type 2 diabetes, ongoing inflammation, constant thirst, headaches, and other complications.

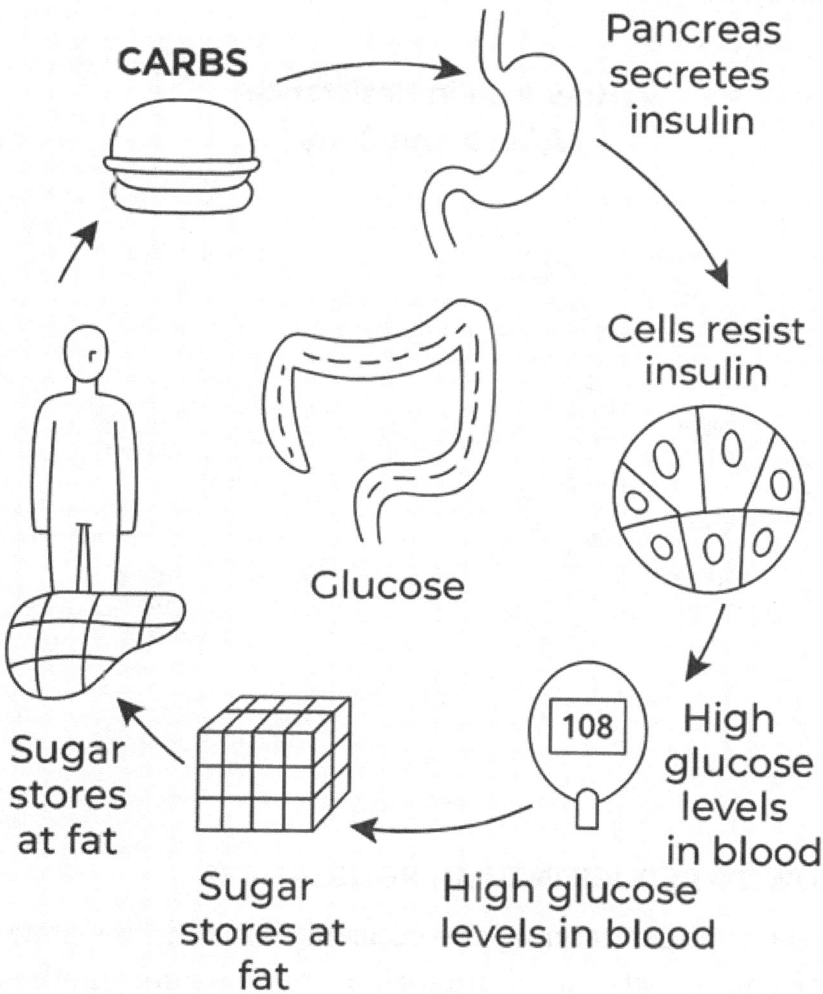

The good news is this process can be reversed. With the right changes in diet such as cut down on sugar and high carbohydrate consumption, movement, stress management, and sleep, your cells can "open their doors" again and begin responding to insulin more effectively. Step by step, you can lower insulin resistance, restore your energy, and protect your long-term health.

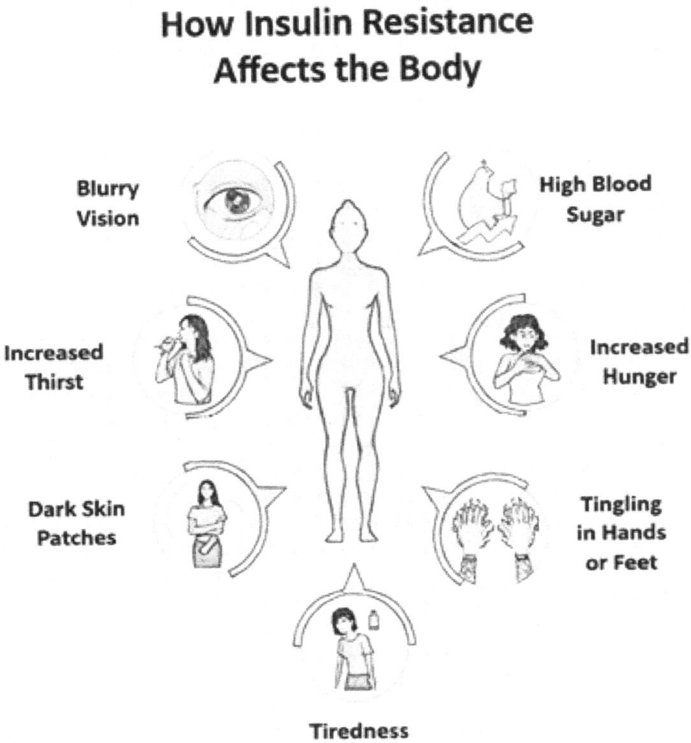

HOW TO REDUCE INSULIN RESISTANCE?

After understanding the concept of insulin resistance and its effects, it is important to consider methods for addressing it. Reducing sugar consumption and increasing physical activity are factors that can influence insulin sensitivity. Both exercise and certain medications also help enhance insulin sensitivity.

As we exercise, our muscles use sugar as an energy source. Glucose is the only form of sugar that can be used as an immediate energy source. The body utilizes stored glycogen and fat as energy sources. It converts it into sugar to meet the demand for energy and glucose in muscle cells.

Glucose is stored in the form of glycogen in liver and muscle cells. Muscles use both glucose and glycogen during exercise, depending upon the intensity and duration. Muscles use glycogen for immediate and primary source at the start of exercise when glycogen is broken down to glucose. During prolonged and lower intensity exercise blood glucose is used as energy source. Insulin levels go down and make it easier to release glucose from the liver. This can further help with the fatty liver disease.

Metformin is commonly prescribed as the initial treatment for diabetes because it reduces insulin resistance. Insulin resistance can also lead to polycystic ovarian syndrome (PCOS), which will be explained further in the women's health section. Metformin is recommended for patients with PCOS as well.

3. Obstructive sleep apnea (OSA)

Once we had a patient in our practice, a 46-year-old engineer, who was always healthy and active until in his mid-30s. Slowly he more sedentary, and with bad dietary choices and he started gaining weight. Before he realized, he was already over 400 pounds. He was more fatigued during the daytime, had difficulty concentrating and not feeling refreshed in the morning. At first, he shrugged it off as just getting older. But when he started nodding off during meetings at work and had frequent episodes of gasping for air at night, he decided to see his doctor. After describing his symptoms and undergoing a sleep study, he was diagnosed with obstructive sleep apnea.

Unfortunately, due to a lack of available CPAP machines during the recent pandemic era, he was unable to obtain his device in a timely manner.

Despite this, he worked diligently on his weight management and managed to lose nearly 70 pounds. He eventually underwent the bariatric procedure, but afterwards developed atrial fibrillation, a heart condition linked to untreated sleep apnea.

If you are dealing with obesity and feeling extremely tired during the day, along with excessive snoring at night, there is a chance that you might be suffering from obstructive sleep apnea. This condition involves multiple episodes where breathing stops for a few seconds during the night. This interferes with the oxygen supply to the brain. As a result, you may suddenly wake up, gasping for breath.

Screening for sleep apnea in a clinical setting can be conducted through a series of targeted questions. Following this initial assessment, individuals may be referred for an official sleep study program to confirm the diagnosis. Sleep apnea is most commonly treated with CPAP. The other options include positional therapy, oral appliances and surgical options like uvulopalatoplasty, nasal surgery and Inspire therapy (nerve stimulator). Weight loss remains the main treatment. Notably, a reduction of as little as 5% of one's baseline weight can significantly alleviate the symptoms associated with sleep apnea. It has been observed that individuals who achieve weight loss may no longer require Continuous Positive Airway Pressure (CPAP) therapy.

It is important to emphasize the necessity of using a CPAP (Continuous Positive Airway Pressure) machine at night if you have sleep apnea. Failing to do so can place excessive stress on the heart and lead to various complications. This is especially crucial for individuals considering bariatric surgery.

The outcome was positive for our patient, as he has since lost 200 pounds. This experience highlighted the importance of consistent use of the CPAP machine before and after bariatric surgery. Six months later, a repeat sleep study showed no signs of sleep apnea, indicating that effective weight loss resolved his condition.

It is crucial to acknowledge that many patients are unable to use CPAP due to their intolerance to the masks or the pressures exerted by these machines. Long-term non-adherence rates to PAP devices can reach as high as 60-70% among patients, leading to heightened cardiovascular and neurological disease risks. Therefore, implementing an effective weight management strategy is particularly important for this population.

Quality sleep is just as crucial to your health as maintaining a balanced diet and engaging in regular exercise. When sleep is disrupted, it can interfere with the hormones that regulate appetite, cravings, and metabolism, which in turn makes weight management more challenging. Prioritizing good sleep habits allows your body to recover, helps to balance hormone levels, increases energy, and strengthens your overall health.

To support healthy sleep, consider implementing the following:

- **Stick to a schedule:** Go to bed and wake up at the same time every day, including weekends. Consistency helps regulate your body's internal clock, promoting better sleep quality.
- **Limit screens before bed:** Turn off personal devices and TVs at least an hour before going to sleep. Reducing screen time in the evening can help your mind wind down and prepare for restful sleep.
- **Create a calm environment:** Make your bedroom cool, quiet, and dark. This can eliminate distractions and enhance your sleep setting.
- **Watch what you eat and drink:** Avoid consuming caffeine, alcohol, and heavy meals close to bedtime, as these can disrupt your sleep cycle and make it harder to fall asleep.
- **Build a wind-down routine:** Incorporate relaxing activities such as reading, light stretching, or meditation before bed to signal to your body that it's time to rest.
- **Get morning light:** Exposure to natural light early in the day helps reset your circadian rhythm, making it easier to fall asleep at night and wake up in the morning.
- **Reserve your bed for sleep:** Use your bed only for sleep and intimacy, avoiding work, scrolling on devices,

or watching TV in bed, to reinforce the connection between your bed and sleep.

By consistently applying these strategies, you can improve your sleep quality, which will support your physical health and help you more effectively manage your weight.

4. Hypertension

High blood pressure (BP) is commonly linked to weight gain, with a particularly strong association in individuals who have sleep apnea and among younger age groups. In these populations, high blood pressure often presents as diastolic hypertension, which means that the lower number in a blood pressure reading is elevated.

Weight gain can lead to an increase in blood pressure through several mechanisms. First, it results in increased sodium absorption by the body, which can contribute to higher blood volume and elevated blood pressure. Additionally, weight gain stimulates the sympathetic nervous system, causing the heart and blood vessels to work harder.

Another important factor is the activation of the Renin-Angiotensin-Aldosterone System (RAAS) in the kidneys. This system plays a central role in regulating blood pressure by controlling blood vessel constriction and the balance of fluids and salts in the body. When activated by excess weight, it can lead to further increases in blood pressure.

The good news is that losing as little as 5% of your baseline body weight can lower your blood pressure by approximately 10 points. This improvement highlights the significant impact that even modest weight loss can have on your cardiovascular health.

5. Diabetes

Gaining weight plays a major role in making people prone to diabetes. It starts with pre-diabetes when hemoglobin A1c is between 5.7 to 6.4, giving rise to high sugar levels due to insulin resistance. This is primarily the result of unhealthy eating habits. Extra sugars and carbohydrates lead to elevated insulin levels and Insulin resistance, as discussed in the insulin resistance section.

People who lose weight by medical or surgical means see a significant improvement in hemoglobin A1c. Research shows that losing as little as 5 to 10% of your body weight triples the chance of lowering your A1c by 0.5.

Weight gain is a significant factor contributing to the development of diabetes. The process often begins with pre-diabetes, which is identified when hemoglobin A1c levels are between 5.7% and 6.2%. In this stage, elevated blood sugar levels arise primarily due to insulin resistance. This resistance is largely the result of unhealthy eating habits, particularly the consumption of excess sugars and carbohydrates. These dietary patterns lead to increased insulin levels in the body, which, over time, cause the cells to become less responsive to insulin's effects.

As discussed in the section on insulin resistance, this progression can be reversed. Individuals who lose weight - whether through medical or surgical methods - often experience meaningful improvements in their hemoglobin A1c levels. **Studies show that losing 5%-10% of body weight may lower hemoglobin A1c by 0.5%.** This demonstrates the powerful impact that even modest weight loss can have on improving blood sugar control and reducing the risk of developing diabetes.

6. Elevated cholesterol

Hyperlipidemia, commonly referred to as high cholesterol, is a condition in which cholesterol accumulates in the bloodstream. Cholesterol itself is a fat-like substance that, when present in excess, can significantly raise the risk of developing heart disease. Notably, heart disease remains the leading cause of death in the United States.

- Each 10 pounds of excess fat produces an additional 10 mg of cholesterol daily.
- Obesity is a common cause of high triglycerides.
- High triglycerides are a common cause of fatty liver disease.
- If left unmanaged, fatty liver disease may progress to more serious conditions, including cirrhosis and, in severe cases, liver failure.

Fortunately, weight loss can have a marked positive effect on cholesterol and triglyceride levels. Research has shown that losing approximately 20 pounds can lead to a

15% reduction in LDL (low-density lipoprotein) cholesterol, a 30% decrease in triglycerides, an increase in HDL (high-density lipoprotein) cholesterol, and an overall reduction in total cholesterol levels. These improvements highlight the crucial role of weight management in promoting cardiovascular and liver health.

7. Polycystic ovarian syndrome (PCOS)

PCOS is a major women's health condition related to weight gain. It is a hormonal imbalance that results from anovulation (inability of the ovaries to make an egg). Ovaries can have multiple fluid-filled cysts called polycystic ovaries. Ovaries make high levels of male hormones called androgens, which lead to excessive facial hair. Conditions affect women of reproductive age. It can cause irregular periods, infertility, excess hair, acne, and weight gain.

Criteria for the diagnosis of PCOS require that two of the three following factors to be present:

- Ovaries with multiple cysts (ultrasound may appear normal)
- Irregular, infrequent, or absent menstrual periods
- Male-pattern hair distribution, physical signs of excess male hormones, or blood tests indicating elevated male hormones

About half of people with PCOS experience insulin resistance, which may lead to infertility, higher risks for type 2 diabetes, heart disease, sleep apnea, stroke, and symptoms of anxiety or depression if untreated.

The first line of action is lifestyle modifications in the form of a healthy diet and regular exercise, which will help in weight loss.

Even a modest reduction in body weight, such as losing just 5%, can lead to significant improvements in the symptoms and underlying issues of polycystic ovarian syndrome (PCOS). This degree of weight loss can help regulate menstrual cycles, decrease insulin resistance, and reduce the severity of symptoms such as excess hair and acne.

In addition to lifestyle modifications, the medication metformin is commonly used as a therapeutic option. Metformin may be prescribed to help address the metabolic abnormalities and symptoms associated with PCOS by improving insulin sensitivity and supporting the management of this condition.

8. Joint pains

Joint pain frequently occurs when there is increased stress placed on the joints, especially as a result of carrying excess body weight. This additional weight acts as a mechanical force, intensifying the pressure on the joints. Over time, this persistent strain can contribute to the development and progression of arthritis. The combination of mechanical stress and inflammation within the joints often leads to ongoing discomfort and further deterioration of joint health.

Losing 1 pound of weight can relieve 4 pounds of excess pressure on the knees.

Managing weight effectively can help alleviate ongoing discomfort and may slow the progression of joint deterioration, making weight loss a key factor in joint health maintenance.

People with arthritis often need knee arthroplasties or joint replacement surgeries. However, the outcome of such surgeries depends on successful weight management prior to those procedures. Even after the successful joint replacement surgery, it is important to continue to maintain a healthy weight to minimize long-term complications. Many insurance companies are now asking for the BMI to be under a certain range before those surgeries can be conducted.

9. Cancer

Obesity is related to the development of 13 kinds of cancers. Overweight and obesity can cause long-lasting inflammation and higher-than-normal levels of insulin, insulin-like growth factor, and sex hormones. These changes may lead to cancer. Breast cancer after menopause is the most common obesity-associated cancer among women. Colorectal cancer is the most common obesity-associated cancer among men. Treatment and prevention of cancer related to obesity again advise consuming a mindful diet, maintaining a healthy lifestyle, increasing physical activity, cutting down on refined sugars and carbohydrates, and losing weight.

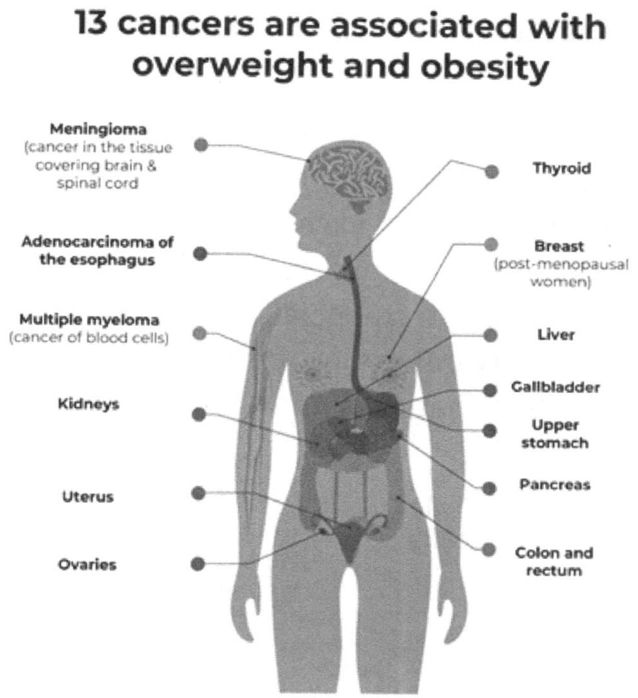

Source: https://stacks.cdc.gov/view/cdc/48491

2.3 OBESITY AS A HIGH INFLAMMATORY STATE

Obesity is not just excess weight - it is a **state of chronic inflammation.** As fat cells **(adipocytes)** grow in number and size, they release chemicals such as cytokines and adipokines that trigger ongoing, low-grade inflammation throughout the body. Unlike the short-term inflammation that helps us heal from injuries, this chronic form lingers and can damage blood vessels, organs, and joints.

This inflammation is strongly linked to insulin resistance, heart disease, diabetes, and even certain cancers. There is significant ongoing research on the ways to reduce it.

Even social media is filled with anecdotes on the obesity-inflammation connection. Across various platforms, individuals share personal experiences and observations about how excess weight contributes to persistent inflammation and related health issues. The widespread discussion in social media underscores the growing public awareness of the link between obesity and chronic inflammation.

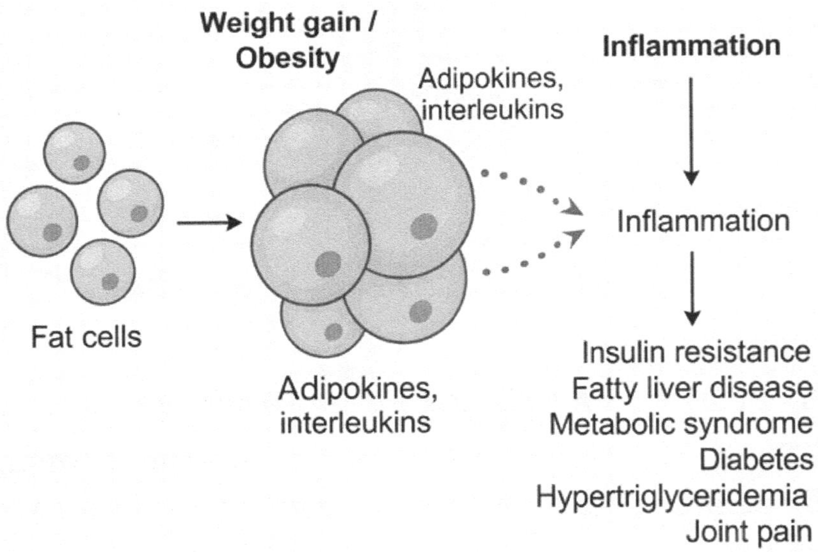

As you can see in the above picture, we gain weight in the form of fat cells. As they increase in number as well as in size, they start releasing certain chemicals called adipokines and interleukins. These chemicals cause inflammation, insulin resistance, fatty liver disease, and metabolic syndrome. The consequence of high inflammation in the body leads to joint pains, aches, fatty liver disease, diabetes, hypertriglyceridemia, and metabolic syndrome.

Certain foods can increase inflammation. There are 4 main characteristics of diet that can be considered anti-inflammatory in nature:

- A diet that is least processed.
- A more natural diet.
- A diet that is not loaded with sugar and carbohydrates.
- A diet rich in polyphenols can help fight inflammation. Fruits, berries, vegetables, whole grains, turmeric, ginger, dark chocolate, nuts, seeds, beans, olive oil, etc., are rich in polyphenols.

Following is a list of some foods that are considered to be highly inflammatory. You can start eliminating those food items from your diet. An anti-inflammatory diet is often advised for fatty liver disease.

Foods that cause inflammation (As per Harvard Health)

Try to avoid or limit these foods as much as possible:

- Refined carbohydrates, such as white bread and pastries.
- French fries and other fried foods.
- Soda and other sugar-sweetened beverages.
- Red meat (burgers, steaks) and processed meat (hot dogs, sausage).

- Margarine, shortening, and lard.

Anti-inflammatory foods

An anti-inflammatory diet should include these foods:

- Olive oil.
- Green leafy vegetables, such as spinach, kale, and collards.
- Nuts like almonds and walnuts.
- Fatty fish, like salmon, mackerel, tuna, and sardines.
- Fruits such as strawberries, blueberries, cherries, and oranges.

Scan the above-given QR code to know more about the anti-inflammatory diet from Harvard Health.

Please read this thoroughly to understand the quality or efficacy of your daily consumption. Even if you are dealing with weight issues, an anti-inflammatory diet in general is good for people experiencing generalized body aches, pains, rheumatologic conditions, and feeling tired all day. An anti-inflammatory diet plays a big role in improving overall health.

Anti-inflammatory

Foods to Eat

Vegetables

- Leafy greens (spinach, kale, Swiss chard, collard greens)
- Cauliflower and Broccoli
- Beetroot
- Asparagus
- Garlic and Onions
- Radishes
- Bell Peppers (red, yellow, green)
- Celery
- Tomatoes
- Brussels Sprouts
- Carrots
- Cabbage
- Artichokes and Eggplant
- Leeks
- Zucchini
- Turnips
- Radishes

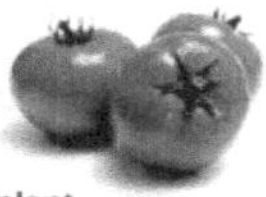

Fish

- Sardines
- Herring Anchovies
- Tilapia
- Tuna
- Salmon
- Trout
- Mackerel
- Cod
- Halibut

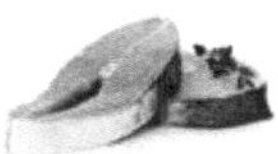

Meats and Proteins

- Lean Poultry (chicken breast, turkey breast)
- Eggs (preferably free-range or omega-3 enriched)
- Edamame
- Skinless Turkey or Chicken Legs
- Tofu
- Bison
- Grass-fed beef/lamb
- Tempeh

Nuts and Seeds

- Almonds
- Walnuts
- Sesame Seeds
- Cashews
- Flaxseeds
- Pecans
- Chia Seeds
- Sunflower Seeds
- Pumpkin Seeds

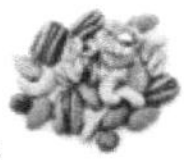

Whole Grains

- Brown Rice
- Buckwheat
- Farro Bulgur Amaranth
- Whole Wheat
- Oats
- Quinoa Barley
- Millet

Herbs & Spices

- Garlic Cinnamon
- Cayenne Pepper
- Basil
- Thyme
- Turmeric
- Ginger
- Black Pepper Cloves
- Rosemary

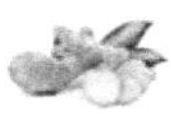

Fruits

- Berries
- Watermelon
- Papaya
- Pineapple
- Oranges
- Kiwi
- Apples
- Grapes
- Pears

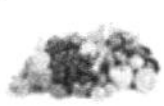

Healthy Fats

- Extra Virgin Olive Oil
- Flaxseed Oil
- Walnut Oil
- Chia seeds
- Olives
- Almond Butter
- Avocado Oil
- Coconut Oil
- Cashew Butter
- Hemp Seeds

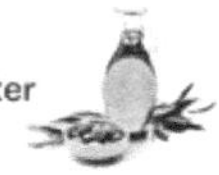

Beverages

- Chamomile or Peppermint
- Water infused with Cucumber and Lemon
- Pineapple Juice
- Matcha Tea
- Green Tea
- Turmeric Milk
- Ginger Tea
- Turmeric Latte made with almond/coconut milk
- Beet Juice

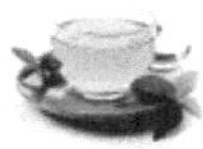

Condiments

- Olive Oil
- Apple Cider Vinegar
- Balsamic Vinegar
- Hummus
- Green Pesto
- Tahini
- Miso Paste
- Lemon Juice
- Mustard (whole grain)
- Soy Sauce (low sodium or tamari)

Fermented Foods

- Kimchi
- Kefir
- Yogurt
- Sauerkraut

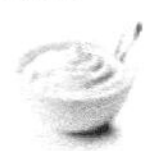

Foods to Avoid

Sugary Foods and Beverages

- Soda
- Chocolate with high sugar content
- Fruit Juices with added sugar
- Candy Bars
- Sweetened Iced Tea

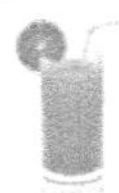

Trans Fats and Unhealthy Fats

- Deep-fried foods
- Processed Snacks
- Store-bought pie crusts and doughs
- Margarine
- Vegetable shortening

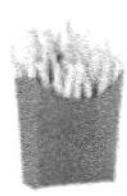

Processed Foods

- Fast food (burgers, fries, chicken nuggets)
- Corned beef
- Convenience foods (instant noodles, canned pasta, etc)
- Hot Dogs
- Frozen Meals (pizza, lasagna)
- Packaged Snacks (chips, cheese puffs, etc)

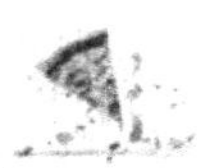

Refined Carbohydrates

- White Bread
- Pastries
- Pasta made with refined flour
- Breakfast Cereal
- White Rice

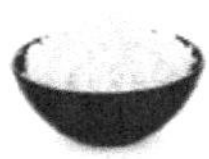

Foods High in Refined Sugars

- Desserts (cakes, pies, etc)
- Pastries
- Flavoured Yogurt with added sugar
- Breakfast cereals with added sugar
- Sugary snacks (gummy candies, sweetened granola bars)

Dairy Products

- Cream
- Whole milk
- Flavoured yogurt
- Sweetened Condensed Milk
- Full-fat yogurt
- Cheese
- Full-fat sour cream
- Margarine

Omega-6 Rich Oils

- Cottonseed oil
- Sunflower Oil
- Safflower Oil
- Soybean oil
- Corn oil

High- saturated fat foods

- Fatty cuts of meat
- Processed meats
- Butter
- Palm Oil
- Full-fat dairy products

High-sodium foods

- Canned soups
- Pickles
- Salted nuts and seeds
- Processed meats
- Canned vegetables with added salt

High-Glycemic Index Foods

- White Pasta
- Bagels
- Instant Oatmeal
- Condensed Milk
- Instant Rice
- Cornflakes
- Puffed rice cereal
- Pretzels
- Cream Cheese
- Buttermilk
- White Bread
- Instant Oatmeal
- Instant mashed potatoes
- Rice cakes
- White Rice

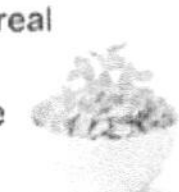

Excessive Alcohol

- Beer
- Wine Spirits (vodka, whiskey, rum)
- Cocktails with sugary misers
- Liqueurs

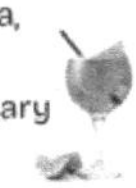

Nightshade Vegetables

- Eggplant
- Bell peppers (red, green, yellow)
- White potatoes
- Tomatillos
- Paprika Pimentos

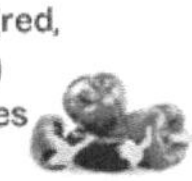

2.4 MYTHS ABOUT OBESITY

1. Weight gain due to lack of willpower and motivation:

Weight gain is often related more to our environment than just our willpower. If we cultivate self-discipline and consistency while taking care of our surroundings, we can be more successful in our weight loss journey. Additionally, various hormones play a role in regulating metabolism.

2. Intense workouts are necessary for weight loss:

The belief that we must work hard and engage in intense workouts to lose weight can sometimes be a setback that prevents us from starting our journey. Instead, beginning with a simple routine, like walking for 10 minutes after each meal, can prove to be extremely beneficial. Setting realistic goals can make the process feel less daunting.

3. The need to starve or skip meals to lose weight:

Skipping meals or eating too few calories can lower our metabolism, which ultimately slows down our weight loss journey. Consuming 3 meals a day with a balanced amount of carbohydrates, fruits, and vegetables in appropriate portion sizes could be more effective than randomly skipping meals or avoiding food altogether.

4. Walking for long hours can be a good workout option:

While walking is excellent for maintaining health and reducing stress, it may not be sufficient for those actively trying to lose weight. However, walking is a great starting point for individuals who have never exercised before. Low-intensity walking alone may not effectively target fat loss, which requires a higher level of intensity in workouts. Though shorter, these high-intensity workouts are essential for burning fat. It is important to remember that walking is always a good first step, especially if you have been sedentary for long periods of time.

5. Bariatric surgery is an easy solution:

Bariatric surgery may seem like a quick fix solution to achieve weight loss, especially in patients with a very high BMI, who have not had any success with conservative measures. However, it is vital to understand that surgery should never be viewed as an easy solution. To achieve lasting results after bariatric surgery, the patients must still focus on being disciplined and making lifestyle changes.

Now that we have addressed the basic aspects and causes of obesity, let us discuss the treatment part.

FOUR LEGS OF OBESITY MANAGEMENT CHAIR:

This journey can be conceptualized as a chair supported by 4 legs, with each individually representing diet, exercise, behavior, and medications. In this book, I will address each of these components in detail.

Diet serves as the foremost aspect that requires our attention. By exploring this element thoroughly, readers will gain a comprehensive understanding of its significance and impact. We'll cover all four pillars one by one, starting with behavior. Understanding the mindset behind an eating habit can certainly help with better food choices and make us more receptive to change.

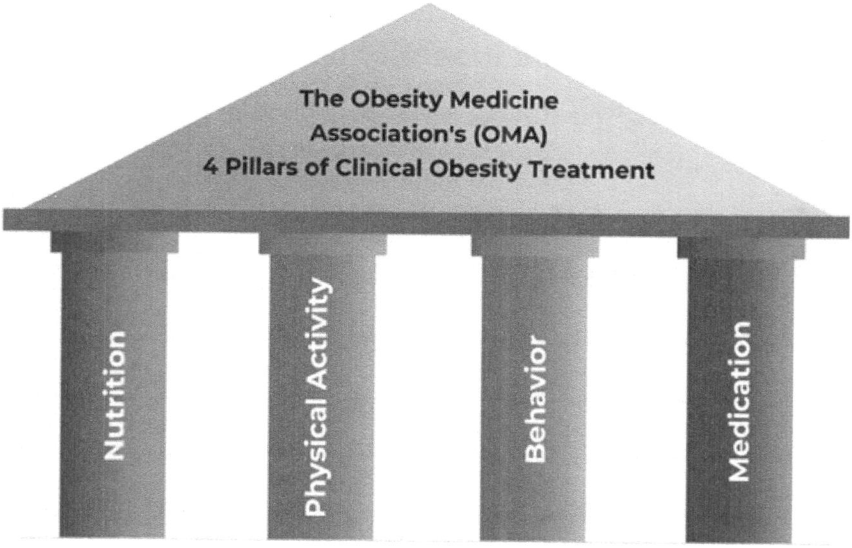

ABC Technique

A - Awareness → B - Behavior → C - Change

A - Awareness: Understanding Obesity

"You can't change what you don't understand."

Obesity is a complex medical condition that involves more than just numbers such as BMI, waist circumference, or body composition. Its root causes are diverse, including biological factors like genetics, metabolism, and hormones such as insulin, leptin, etc; behavioral aspects like inactivity, emotional eating, and poor sleep; as well as environmental influences such as food marketing, processed foods, and chronic stress. The health consequences can be significant, leading to inflammation, insulin resistance, cardiovascular disease, sleep apnea, arthritis, cancer etc. It's important to understand that obesity is not a failure of willpower, but a complex health condition very often clouded by stigma and misconceptions.

Reflections

- What's your personal understanding of obesity?

___

___

___

___

- Have you ever been blamed or judged for your weight?

___

___

___

___

- What influences your eating and activity patterns the most?

___

___

___

___

B - Behavior: Identifying Habit Loops

"Behavior is the bridge between knowing and doing."

Take time to examine your daily behaviors, routines, and coping mechanisms that may contribute to weight gain or prevent weight loss. **Habit Formation:** Cue → Craving → Response → Reward (based on the concept of behavior loops).

Examine your daily behaviors, routines, and coping mechanisms that contribute to weight gain or prevent weight loss. Habits often follow a pattern of cue, craving, response, and reward, and recognizing these behavior loops can be transformative. For instance, eating in response to stress may bring short-term relief but can lead to long-term regret, while skipping meals might prompt overeating later and create a cycle of fatigue. Common behaviors linked to obesity include mindless eating, consuming sugar-sweetened beverages, nighttime snacking, and physical inactivity. To build awareness, tools like food journals, mood-hunger-behavior logs, or wearable trackers (monitoring steps, sleep, and more) can provide important insights and help you observe your patterns more objectively.

Reflections

- What behaviors do I notice that may be holding me back?

- When am I most vulnerable to overeating or skipping activity?

- What's one small behavior I can observe, not judge?

C - Change: Building a Healthier Pattern

"Change doesn't require perfection - it requires intention."

Instead of focusing solely on weight loss, try shifting your goal toward overall health gains by making small, sustainable changes. For example, consider adding a ten-minute walk to your daily routine, incorporating more vegetables into your meals, or reducing screen time at night. Track your progress in ways that go beyond the scale - notice improvements in your mood, energy, and mobility. Celebrate these positive changes and start to see yourself as someone who prioritizes health. By embracing this identity shift, you can foster a mindset that supports lasting well-being rather than simply fixating on the numbers.

Reflections:

- What change feels doable this week?

____

____

____

____

- What's a recent win, even if small?

____

____

____

____

- How do I want to define success on this journey?

____

____

____

____

Chapter : 3

Behavior and Mindset

"We are what we repeatedly do. Excellence, then, is not an act, but a habit."

-Aristotle

THE MIND SHIFT

There was a little boy who was deeply passionate about chess. Yet no matter how hard he tried, he never seemed to secure a victory. Frustrated, he approached his dad and asked, "Why can't I win despite trying my best?" His dad paused thoughtfully for a moment, looked him in the eyes, and simply asked, "Whom are you playing against?"

The boy replied peevishly, "Myself!" It became clear that he was competing against his own mind, wrestling with his thoughts and doubts.

This scenario is quite similar to the weight loss journey. In both cases, we often find ourselves battling against our own minds and struggling to overcome internal barriers. Mindset is the most crucial pillar of this journey. It is the foundation that empowers us to push through challenges and work against our own limitations.

Moreover, mindset plays a vital role in weight maintenance after achieving weight loss. When we prescribe medications for weight management, many people voice their concerns about regaining weight once they stop taking them. We always emphasize that during their time on the medications, they must focus on cultivating a strong mindset and developing healthy habits. This proactive approach ensures that their weight loss is not only successful but also sustainable in the long run.

How does our mind work and form a habit, and what can be done to break it? Let us first understand what exactly this mindset is.

3.1 HOW ARE OUR HABITS FORMED?

Our brain is a remarkable organ, composed of approximately 86 billion neurons, which are specialized cells that transmit information throughout the body. These neurons create communication by firing electrical signals and releasing neurotransmitters, i.e., chemicals that facilitate the exchange of information among them. With repeated use, certain neuron pathways strengthen, leading to the formation of memories, primarily within the limbic system, a key region associated with emotions and memory processing.

Let me explain this in simpler words. Imagine a big grassy park in your neighborhood. People need to cross it to get from one side to the other. At first, everyone chooses their own direction, but eventually most people start taking the same shortcut because it's quicker and easier. After a while, the grass wears down and a visible dirt path forms.

Your brain works in a similar way. The park is your brain, your thoughts are the people walking, and the path is the neural pathway. The more you use the same thought or behavior, the stronger and more automatic that path becomes.

Another way to think of it is your daily commute. If you drive to work the same way every day, the route becomes second nature - you don't even have to think about it. Or think about your phone habits: opening the same app without even realizing it. That's your brain following a well-worn pathway.

Now consider an example involving food. Suppose you try a new dish, which happens to be a rich, creamy chocolate mousse for the first time. Chances are, you will find it utterly delicious. Your brain instantly records this pleasurable experience. The neurons activated during this moment create a vivid mental reel that captures not just the taste, but also the scent, texture, and the joy of eating it. Thus, the next time you encounter this dessert again, your brain automatically replays that same mental reel and the delightful sensations associated with it. This potentially sparks a craving for that dessert.

The good news is that just like you can step off the trail in the park or take a new road to work, you can also create new neural pathways. It takes effort at first, but with repetition, those new paths get stronger, while the old ones fade. That's how real, lasting change happens.

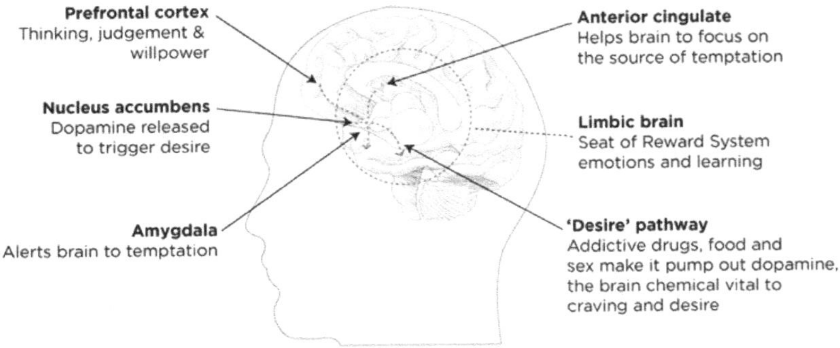

This picture illustrates different areas of the brain and how memories are created.

Take a moment to reflect and write down a few specific foods that you find irresistible, even after enjoying a satisfying meal. Try to remember the flavors or dishes that linger in your memory and tempt you time and again.

____

____

____

____

NATURE OF FOOD THAT FORMS A CRAVING

Have you ever thought why you crave foods like cake, ice cream, and pizza, more than say broccoli or Brussels sprouts? Unhealthy foods are undeniably addictive, while healthier options rarely evoke similar cravings. This is because of the unique properties of these indulgent foods, which trigger the release of dopamine. This is a key chemical in the brain associated with pleasure. Foods that are high in sugar and fat, easy to consume, and possess a high glycemic index are particularly effective in creating cravings. They cause a gush of dopamine in our brain while simultaneously creating a memory associated with that particular food.

The immediate gratification of these delectable treats, which literally melt in your mouth, makes them irresistible. Cravings typically arise from foods rich in fat, refined sugars, and carbohydrates, while invariably lacking in fiber. These high glycemic foods produce a rapid spike in blood sugar levels, further reinforcing the desire for them.

For those who want to delve deeper, Section 7.4 provides comprehensive information on the glycemic index of various foods. This resource will empower you to evaluate your favorite foods based on their glycemic impact. It will help you make informed choices about what you eat.

3.2 FOOD ADDICTION

In the 1950s, scientists conducted an important experiment with rats. They placed electrodes in the rats' brains to release dopamine, a chemical that makes animals feel pleasure. The rats learned to press a lever to get a strong burst of dopamine. They became so focused on pressing the lever that they stopped eating, drinking, and reproducing. All they did was press the lever. Even when scientists connected the lever to an electric shock, the rats continued to press it, ignoring the pain. Such was their addiction to pleasure.

The Link Between Dopamine and Repetitive Behaviors

This research demonstrates a significant relationship between dopamine release and the repetition of certain behaviors. When an activity triggers the release of dopamine, the brain registers it as pleasurable, which in turn encourages individuals to repeat the behavior. This process is not limited to one specific activity; instead, it extends to various experiences that stimulate dopamine production, such as eating food, taking drugs, consuming sugar, achieving goals, engaging in sexual activity, and using social media. Each of these can become recurrent patterns, driven by the brain's natural response to dopamine release.

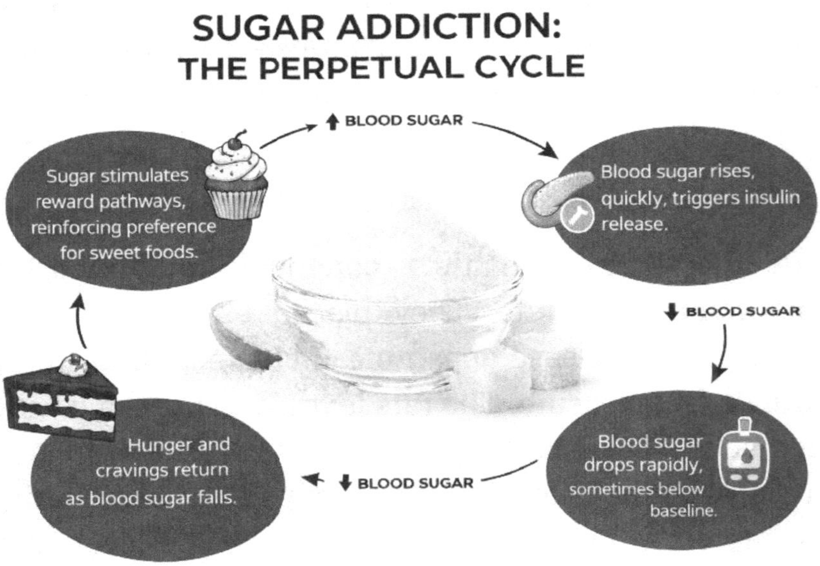

Thus, the main issue is our instinct to seek dopamine. We can better identify these behaviors by understanding what addiction is. We offer tools to help people break free from these patterns and reclaim control over their lives.

3.3 BINGE EATING

The term binge eating is often used loosely, but it involves specific criteria to make it a clinical diagnosis. For example, eating an extra piece of cake after a meal typically wouldn't qualify as binge eating behavior. To accurately diagnose a binge eating disorder, medical and psychological societies have established guidelines that help identify the behavior. Understanding these criteria is essential for recognizing and addressing the issue appropriately.

Diagnostic Criteria for Binge Eating Disorder

- **Recurrent binge eating episodes, defined by:**
  - Eating, in a short period (e.g., within 2 hours), an amount of food that is definitely larger than most people would eat in similar circumstances.
  - Feeling a lack of control during the episode (e.g., can't stop eating, can't control what or how much is eaten).
- **Episodes are associated with at least 3 of the following:**
  - Eating much more rapidly than normal
  - Eating until uncomfortably full
  - Eating large amounts when not physically hungry

- o Eating alone because of embarrassment
- o Feeling disgusted, depressed, or very guilty afterward

- **Marked distress** regarding binge eating is present.
- **Frequency:** Binge eating occurs **at least once a week for 3 months.**
- **Not associated with compensatory behaviors** such as vomiting, excessive exercise, or misuse of laxatives/ diuretics (which would indicate bulimia nervosa instead).

Please visit the link below to take a test on binge eating. Answer the simple questions to the best of your ability. The results will indicate a fairly accurate diagnosis.

Scan the above QR code to know more about binge eating from Psychology Tools.

3.4 CRAVINGS AND EMOTIONS:

Scientific research shows that people who have difficulty expressing their emotions are more prone to binge eating.

Rather than expressing our emotions, we sometimes tend to stuff them down with food that we find comfortable and soothing. Our mind stores that memory to ease out a particular emotion and tends to fire the neuron to seek the same food that leads to a specific craving.

Understanding your cravings can provide valuable insights into your emotions. Each craving often reflects a specific emotional need related to a certain food. Let us do this to gain more insight. Check out common cravings below and see if they meet your underlined emotion.

- **Bread and butter** - may indicate a feeling of being stuck and a desire to make necessary changes.
- **Crisps** - could suggest a need to alleviate anxiety and stress.
- **Chocolate** - often symbolizes a longing for love and affection.
- **Cheese** - might reflect feelings of exhaustion, fear, and a desire for comfort.
- **Coffee** - can point to feelings of burnout and dissatisfaction with your job.
- **Vanilla** - often relates to a desire for fulfillment and renewal in your life.
- **Nuts** - may signify a need for peace of mind amidst stress.

ACTIONABLE STEPS:

Here is a practical stepwise approach to deal with

cravings. Remember, it takes time and practice to be included in the daily routine.

Whenever you experience a strong craving, take a moment to pause and hydrate yourself with a tall glass of water. As you sit back and reflect, ask yourself, "Am I genuinely hungry, or am I simply experiencing a craving? Dig deeper to distinguish between true physical hunger and an emotional longing that leads to these cravings.

Secondly, recognize the specific foods you desire along with the emotions attached to them. This process can reveal insights into your subconscious mind, where you might be avoiding some important issues or feelings that require your attention. For instance, if you are craving a scoop of rich, creamy ice cream, consider whether it stems from a particularly stressful day. You might be subconsciously seeking comfort or consolation as a way to rejuvenate yourself after dealing with challenges.

If you find that you are reaching for chocolate ever so often, it could indicate a deeper yearning for affection or connection. During such moments, it might be helpful to pick up the phone and call a loved one to share some warmth and love.

On the other hand, if your craving leans towards something crispy or crunchy, it may be a manifestation of underlying emotions like anger or frustration. It is important to remember that these feelings are neither good nor bad. Avoid judging yourself for what you feel. Instead, simply acknowledge the underlying emotions. Label them if that helps, and then explore constructive ways to address the root cause behind them. This self-awareness can lead to healthier choices and emotional well-being.

3.5 BOREDOM EATING:

Boredom eating is to fill the void or a sense of emptiness within ourselves due to a lack of engaging activity or motivation. Void can also arise from feelings of dissatisfaction in our lives, particularly when we don't feel valued or appreciated in our personal lives or work environments. It's common to seek comfort in food during these challenging times, but this behavior can lead to a cycle of negative emotions, such as guilt or frustration. Acknowledging this pattern is a courageous first step toward embracing healthier habits.

Here are some simple ways to deal with it. When you find yourself overwhelmed by stress, boredom, anxiety, or anger, it is crucial to explore specific and manageable activities that can serve as a positive outlet. Rather than feeling pressured to engage in intense workouts, consider the calming practice of journaling. It allows you to pour out your thoughts and feelings and can be incredibly therapeutic. Sometimes we tend to carry too much burden in our brains. Noting it down on a piece of paper could be the first step to lighten it.

Another effective strategy is to take a stroll outside, allowing fresh air and the sounds of nature to soothe your mind. You could enhance this experience by listening to your favorite music or podcast that inspires you. Engaging in gentle forms of exercise such as yoga or meditation can also be highly beneficial for your mental well-being. These practices encourage mindfulness and can help center your thoughts.

Engaging in an activity that you like could be a hobby or a passion, like writing, crafting, or even cooking. I have seen in my practice some women engage in house cleaning, which reflects decluttering their lives outside and inside, leaving a more organized and pleasant living environment.

Thanks to advanced technology including AI, nowadays all the wonderful books are available on audio. Listening to your favorite book or a topic related to your interest while doing chores can enrich the mind and prevent you from eating.

Engaging in activities that are not only helpful for this journey but also very relaxing, like baking with whole grains, can help you have healthy snacks at the end.

Most importantly, make those activities a part of your routine. Remember, you are not alone in navigating these feelings. Finding supportive and enjoyable ways to cope can lead to lasting positive changes in your life.

3.6 ACTIONABLE PLAN/ MINDFUL EATING:

"Write every bite." Journaling is an indistinct part of this journey. A food diary is not just a record. It is a journey to deeper self-awareness and healthier choices. By tracking what you consume, you unlock the hidden aspects of your relationship with food, discover emotions behind the food choices, and pave the way for positive changes. **The habit of counting carbs and calories leaves us with so much knowledge and information that stays with us forever, and we can use it for our friends and family.**

Following is an outline to maintain your food diary and mindful eating:

- Capture your daily food intake
- Each morsel you eat deserves recognition. Make it a habit to write down every snack and meal.
- Reflect on feelings and circumstances surrounding eating
- As you write, consider the emotions and situations that accompany your meals. Are you eating out of joy, stress, or habit? This reflection is key to understanding your choices
- Discover foods that fuel mindless eating
- Pay attention to the portion size
- Pay attention to flavors, textures, and aromas to make each bite an experience of its own
- Incorporate practices like slowing down, chewing thoughtfully, and appreciating the food's journey from source to plate
- Eliminating distractions, like watching TV or eating in front of the computer
- Create a serene spot to have your meals in a designated space. Embrace stillness and allow a mindful,

uninterrupted dining experience

Embrace the power of self-encouragement:

- Speak to yourself with kindness
- Consciously practice positive self-talk techniques
- Reframe self-doubt with uplifting affirmations
- Embrace setbacks as learning opportunities
- Instead of viewing setbacks as failures, regard them as valuable lessons on your journey to healthier habits

Conclusion

As you reflect on your relationship with food, let mindfulness and self-awareness guide you towards more intentional choices. Cultivating healthy eating habits is not a destination, but an ever-evolving journey filled with moments of growth, discovery, and joy while eating.

As mentioned earlier, we are so conscious about what clothes we wear. We are picky about our shoes as well. Why don't we become equally mindful about the food that goes inside our bodies and becomes a part of us?

3.7 GOAL SETTING

You are likely familiar with SMART goals, and here is why they matter. If you leave your house without a clear destination, the chances of reaching where you wish to go are slim. This principle applies to every aspect of life.

Clarity about your goals is essential for success.

Take a moment to reflect. Whether you write it down or visualize it, identify your goal. It could be any of the following:

- I want to lose 50 pounds.
- I want to become healthier.
- I want to eliminate my fatty liver disease.
- I want to manage my blood sugar.
- I want to play more with my kids or grandkids.

These are common goals I frequently encounter. It is crucial to distinguish whether this is a genuine goal or just a passing wish.

A wish comes from the heart, whereas a goal is driven by both the mind and the heart. You might wish for something while you sleep, but a true goal is the force that keeps you awake at night, pushing you to take action. Wishing to become wealthy is one thing, but without a solid plan, it remains just that... a wish. In essence, a goal is a wish backed by a concrete plan.

Now, consider your weight. Is it just a wish, or is it a definitive goal? This journey is about transforming your wish into a concrete goal. We are here to provide you with the specific guidance you need to make this happen.

Let's get started with this worksheet to kick off your journey towards achieving your goals. You've got this!

SMART Goals:

Specific (S):

You need to outline specific goals clearly, with what you need to achieve. For example, drinking more water or exercising more cannot be a goal. You want to have a more specific goal. How much weight do you want to lose?

Measurable actions are a blueprint for success.

Define your objective with crystal clarity. Instead of vague aspirations like drink more water or exercise more, zero in on precise targets. For example, set a distinct goal such as to lose 10 pounds in three months. By doing this, you create a clear picture of what you want to achieve.

Measurable (M):

Establish criteria to track your progress. This might include quantifying how many ounces of water you consume daily or how many workout sessions you complete each week. Having measurable milestones allows you to celebrate small victories along the way.

Attainable (A):

Ensure that your goals are achievable and grounded in reality. While ambition is vital, setting yourself up for success means selecting targets that are realistic based on your current circumstances. Consider your lifestyle, resources, and potential obstacles while crafting these goals.

Relevant (R):

Your goals should align with your broader ambitions and values. Ask yourself if achieving this goal truly matters to you. Will it enrich your life or lead you toward your long-term aspirations? Relevance helps maintain motivation and commitment.

Time-bound (T):

Finally, instill a sense of urgency by assigning a deadline to your goals. Rather than leaving your intentions open-ended, set specific timeframes. For instance, aim to reach your weight loss target by the end of June. This encourages a continuous forward momentum and helps you to stay focused.

Be sure to incorporate all 5 components, i.e., Specific, Measurable, Attainable, Relevant, and Time-bound, into your goals to create a powerful framework that propels you toward success.

Know Your Challenges:

Every goal comes with its own set of challenges, which can sometimes derail progress. However, addressing these obstacles effectively can help you stay on track. For example, after a long day at work, I may make poor choices, but I focus on correcting them without dwelling on mistakes. This mindset allows me to prioritize making healthier decisions moving forward.

It is important to remember that perfection is not the

goal. Making consistent, positive choices is what really counts. Regularly reviewing and reformulating your goals is an effective strategy to maintain focus and motivation.

Additionally, setting specific action steps toward your goals can help clarify your path. Writing down your goals periodically can serve as a helpful reminder of your objectives and keep you accountable as you work towards achieving them.

I BELIEVE I CAN

The key is to believe in effectively addressing any challenges that come our way. We don't have to be perfectionists. When we make a less-than-ideal choice, it is important to focus on learning from it and quickly getting back on track without any unnecessary self-criticism.

Understand the value of periodically writing down your goals, and create a constructive list of action items to help you achieve them.

POSITIVE AND NEGATIVE REWARD SYSTEM:

At both a social and personal level, many of us tend to blame ourselves for unhealthy weight gain—thinking it's simply a matter of weak willpower or poor discipline. But the truth is far more complex. Weight gain is influenced not only by lifestyle choices, but also by powerful molecular and hormonal forces working within the body.

As mentioned earlier in the section on diet, our

brain's reward system plays a central role. Every time we encounter something pleasurable—such as eating a favorite food—our brain releases dopamine, the "feel-good" chemical. This surge of dopamine lights up the reward pathways in the brain, giving us a sense of pleasure and reinforcing the behavior.

What makes this even more powerful is the role of the hippocampus, the part of the brain responsible for learning and memory. The hippocampus stores these rewarding experiences, so the next time we see or smell that food, the brain remembers how good it felt and urges us to repeat the behavior.

The challenge is that this system can become highly addictive. Just like with other rewarding experiences, the brain begins to crave more each time. A small piece of chocolate may no longer feel satisfying—you want two pieces, then three. Over time, this creates a cycle of reinforcement where the brain drives us to eat more, even when our body doesn't actually need the calories.

Understanding this biology is critical: it shifts the narrative from self-blame to self-awareness. You are not weak or lacking discipline—your brain is wired to seek reward. The key is learning how to **retrain these pathways** so that healthier choices become the ones your brain craves.

Setting goals could be the first step towards this journey. We encourage you to prepare a worksheet and review it from time to time.

In recent studies over the past decade or so, a system

known as the anti-reward system has been identified. This small structure, called the habenula, is located in the midbrain, near the base of the neck. Its primary function is to regulate the reward system. When the habenula is stimulated, it can lead to feelings of depression and sadness. If we experience happiness and a sense of accomplishment, but also face disappointments and shortcomings, the activation of the habenula can result in negative emotions.

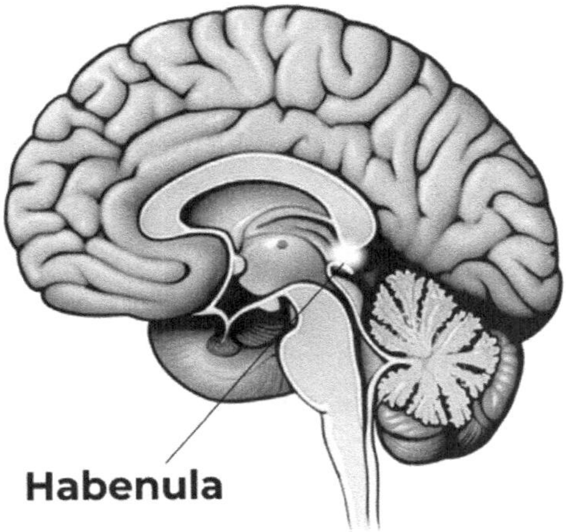

The main reason we struggle to accomplish our SMART goals is that they can lead to disappointment and resentment when we fall short. This feeling can be difficult to overcome at times. Being aware of this can add an additional layer of mindfulness to our goal-setting process.

It is essential to acknowledge that our brains are wired to be significantly more sensitive to loss than to gain, with a responsiveness that is twice as strong.

Therefore, when we fall short of our SMART goals, it is natural to experience feelings of disheartenment and disillusionment. Understanding this dynamic empowers us to navigate setbacks more effectively and reinforces our commitment to achieving our objectives.

ACTIONABLE PLAN:

The antidote to the performance mindset is the iterative mindset. An iterative mindset is characterized by persistence and an acceptance of failure.

Iteration involves repeating actions until we achieve our goals, serving as a remedy for the toxic aspects of a rigid performance mindset. Instead of fixating on strict goals, the iterative mindset encourages us to view failure as a natural part of the learning process, reframing setbacks as opportunities for growth.

To develop an iterative mindset, focus on persistence and be willing to accept mistakes. Embrace your flaws or shortcomings, learn from them, and keep moving forward.

An iterative mindset involves constant observation, analysis, and persistence in making changes. Here are some key characteristics of an iterative mindset:

- **Embrace Mistakes:** Be willing to make mistakes and learn from them. Try to identify unhealthy eating patterns and break them consciously
- **Persistence:** Persistence is a crucial aspect of an iterative mindset. Iteration involves repeating the process with new information. Well begun is half done,

but to get anything done, you are required to persist determinedly

- **View Work and Life as Prototypes:** Both can be continuously improved. Perfection is not a goal, but a pursuit. Even the best you imagine today can be a milestone for something even better. So, keep working on how you can evolve into your best version
- **Focus on the Process:** An iterative mindset emphasizes the process of behavior change rather than just the end product. It involves observing, analyzing, and moving forward.

So let us create a strong platform of mindset for this journey and take this as a principle. Remain persistent in your efforts and willing to learn from your mistakes.

3.8 Cognitive Behavior Therapy (CBT): A Key to Taking Care of Behavior Issues

CBT is a talking therapy used in medical fields that helps people change their behavior, thoughts, and actions. It helps improve medical conditions. It is effective for multiple psychiatric conditions like phobias, eating disorders, depression, anxiety, fear, addiction, etc.

CBT is performed by certified psychiatric counselors. The core values of CBT are as follows:

- Specify a goal
- Identify barriers towards reaching that goal
- Reframe your thinking to get past those barriers

- Practice new behaviors to reinforce new and improved thought patterns

For weight management, CBT is a type of psychotherapy that focuses on the interaction between thoughts, feelings, behaviors, and physical sensations. SMART goals, as discussed above, identify challenges.

Cognitive Behavioral Treatment:

Self-Monitoring

In cognitive behavioral therapy (CBT), you need to watch your behaviors to find triggers that could lead to setbacks. Common triggers include:

- Easy access to high-calorie foods.
- Eating out of boredom or stress.
- Snacking while watching TV.

When you identify a trigger, take action right away. Remove high-calorie foods from your pantry. Stay busy with hobbies. Practice mindfulness to reduce stress. Chew gum while you prepare food, and avoid snacking during TV time.

Catch slip-ups early to protect your progress. Don't fall into a day off mindset. If you really crave for a treat, have just one.

Self-monitoring also means tracking your daily successes. Highlight foods you want to eat more often and set up a workout schedule that includes cardio one day and strength training the next.

Feedback and Reinforcement:

Tracking your food and exercise helps you get feedback. Your therapist will encourage you. Reviewing your logs will show where you can improve and what you should celebrate. Remember, changing your lifestyle takes time. Learn from setbacks and move on.

Positive Attitude:

Be proud of your efforts in this process. Find a mentor who has succeeded. If he can reach their goals, you can too.

Incentives:

Tracking your food and exercise is a part of your incentive plan. While your main goal is to reach your target weight, celebrate small milestones along the way. These small wins will keep you motivated.

ABC Technique:

A - Awareness → B - Behavior → C - Change

A - Awareness: Understanding the Mental and Emotional Drivers

"Awareness is the first act of self-respect."

Become aware - without judgment - of the underlying patterns and psychological triggers that influence your eating behaviors. As noted above, our habits often form through cue, routine, and reward loops, and with repetition, these behaviors become automatic as the brain tends to favor the path of least resistance. Many eating habits are actually triggered by emotional states, environmental cues, or routine timing, rather than genuine hunger. Cravings frequently arise from emotional discomfort, such as stress, loneliness, or anxiety, prompting impulsive eating. Boredom can also drive us to eat, turning food into a source of stimulation or distraction, especially during activities like watching TV or using our phones. Furthermore, highly processed foods can hijack the brain's reward pathways, sometimes leading to patterns of binge eating characterized by a loss of control, feelings of guilt, and shame - a cycle often rooted in unmet emotional needs.

Reflections:

• When do I crave food the most? What underlying emotion might be present?

____

____

____

____

• What is one recurring habit I want to observe and understand, without trying to fix it yet?

____

____

____

____

- What are some non-hunger reasons that prompt me to reach for food?

____

____

____

____

B - Behavior: Mapping Triggers and Building Intentional Routines

"Behavior is where awareness meets decision."

Now we turn our attention to our behaviors, the next step is to map patterns and gradually introduce new micro-actions. Begin by bringing awareness to common cues such as time, place, mood, people, and habitual routines. Develop an actionable plan for mindful eating by pausing before each meal and asking yourself, "Am I truly hungry, or am I experiencing another feeling?" Practice eating without screens, chew slowly, and pay attention to your sense of fullness. Setting SMART goals - those that are Specific, Measurable, Achievable, Relevant, and Time-bound - can support this process. For example, you might decide to "eat at the table three times this week" or "journal for five minutes before snacking." Helpful tools include keeping a craving tracker to note what was happening, what emotions you felt, and how you responded, as well as conducting a behavior chain analysis to observe the sequence from trigger to thought, feeling, action, and result. Exploring mindful substitutions, such as choosing tea instead of snacks when bored, can also foster healthier routines.

Reflections:

- What time, place, or mood usually triggers my unplanned eating?

____

____

____

____

- What's one routine I could slightly adjust to reduce mindless eating?

____

____

____

____

- What's one realistic health goal I can commit to this week?

____

____

____

____

C - Change: Cognitive Rewiring and Long-Term Transformation

"Lasting change comes from changing how you think, not just what you eat."

Change begins when we challenge unhelpful thoughts and reinforce new behaviors - this is the essence of cognitive behavioral therapy (CBT). CBT recognizes that our thoughts influence our emotions, which in turn shape our behaviors; for example, believing "I blew my diet" may lead to feelings of shame and the urge to binge, but reframing that thought as "It was just one choice, not the end" can break the cycle. By identifying cognitive distortions, such as all-or-nothing thinking or catastrophizing, and practicing new scripts like "I can pause," "I'm learning," or "This craving will pass," we nurture healthier habits. Sustaining meaningful change is not about perfection, but about building resilience and gradually adopting the mindset, "I'm someone who cares for my body."

Reflections:

- What thought usually follows a slip or "bad" food choice - and is it helpful?

____

____

____

____

- How can I reframe a slip as a learning opportunity instead of a failure?

___

___

___

___

- Who am I becoming through these small changes? What identity am I stepping into?

___

___

___

___

Chapter : 4

Food/Diet

"Let food be thy medicine and medicine be thy food."

-Hippocrates

WHAT YOU EAT MATTERS - AND WHY

Let us understand the first pillar of weight management by understanding more about calories.

4.1 CALORIE/ CARBS/ FAT

Before we talk about diet, it is important to understand some simple terms that are most commonly used. You must have all heard about calories, BMR, and energy expenditure in some conversation or the other.

Calories

Calorie is a unit of heat energy needed today. It is the temperature of 1 kg of water by 1°C to express in terms of the nutritional value of food. Every food we eat or drink helps produce a certain number of calories that are used to perform activities of daily living.

If we intake more calories than we spend, we tend to gain weight. Depending on the food item, every food has a different caloric value.

In simple terms, 1 g of carbohydrate will produce 4.5 calories, and 1 gram of protein produces the same, while 1 gram of fat leads to the production of 9.5 calories. The body uses these calories to perform daily functions. If not used, these extra calories get converted into fat and are stored in the body.

The exact content of carbohydrates, proteins, and fats will be provided in a separate section to give you an idea while planning your meals.

BMR (Basic Metabolic Rate)

The amount of energy needed while resting is called BMR. It is equivalent to the amount of gas an idle car consumes while parked. On average, it is up to 70% of total energy as compared to 20% of physical activity, and 10% is needed for the digestion of food.

You are constantly burning some energy while resting, even if you are not involved in any exercise-like activity. Obviously, you will burn extra calories while exercising. So, we calculate the basal metabolic rate through a body composition machine or through a formula that is the number of calories you need to maintain your daily weight. BMR varies from person to person depending on age, sex, weight, height, and activity level. We calculate BMR during the first office visit.

Some people have a high metabolic rate. This also depends on the kind of food you consume and the intensity of your activity performance. BMR depends upon muscle mass, age, genetics, diet, and physical activity level.

Hence, the Total Daily Energy Expenditure (TDEE) equates to BMR times activity factor.

Diet Basics

There are 3 fuel tanks in our body.

Your Fuel Tank

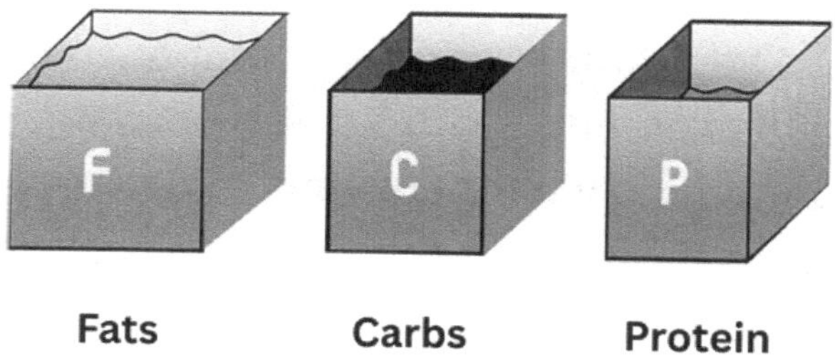

Our body has 3 fuel tanks, i.e., carbohydrates, fats, and proteins. We need energy to perform any activity of daily life. Many of the body cells use carbohydrates as the first energy source before using fats.

A balanced diet consists of all 3 of them in a particular proportion. You need to cut down on carbohydrates to consume a low-carb diet.

Let us talk about individual macronutrients and know good sources. If you are given a particular diet plan by your dietician, you can always refer to the list given below to make it a part of your diet in terms of proteins, carbohydrates, and fats.

4.2 Proteins

Proteins are the building blocks of our body. They are made up of chains of amino acids and are essential for maintaining structure, strength, and function throughout the body. They form essential components such as collagen in bones and skin, keratin in hair, actin and myosin in muscle, as well as enzymes and many hormones that regulate vital functions. For example, glucagon-like peptide-1 (GLP-1), the hormone targeted by medications like semaglutide, is a 41-amino-acid chain that plays a key role in appetite regulation and metabolism.

Because proteins are primarily used for growth, repair, and regulation, they are not the body's main source of energy. There are 7 essential amino acids that our body cannot produce and must be obtained through the diet, making adequate protein intake vital for overall health.

Essential Amino Acids For Humans	
Essential Amino Acids	**Common Sources**
Methionine	Corns, Dairy, Meat, Whole Grains
Lysine	Beans, Lentils, Meat, Spinach
Valine	Dairy, Grains, Meat
Threonine	Dairy, Meat, Nuts, Seeds
Isoleucine	Dairy, Lentils, Meat, Wheat
Leucine	Cottage Cheese, Lentils, Meat, Peanuts
Phenylalanine	Dairy, Meat, Peanuts, Seeds
Tryptophan	Dairy, Meat, Oats

Above is a list of essential amino acids. Meat and dairy are good sources to receive all the essential amino acids.

A few common questions that come to mind about protein are how much protein I should consume on a daily basis.

An average human needs close to 0.8 to 1.2 g of protein per kg. If somebody does intense workouts, the requirement goes up to 2 g per kg.

Usually, we need close to 20-25 g per meal, 3 times a day, and 10-15 g during snacks as well. Remember, proteins cause muscle synthesis, but that trigger goes on only for 3 hours. So, if somebody is athletic and engaged in intense workouts, that signal needs to go on every 3 hours. So, athletes should consume some protein frequently every 3 hours.

What are the best timings to eat protein?

It is advisable to eat protein throughout the day. So, instead of eating 80 g in the morning, it would be better to eat 20 g four times every day.

What happens if I don't have any protein in my diet?

A protein-deficient diet can lead to hair fall, weak bones, poor musculature, and a compromised immunity.

Following is an extensive list of healthy proteins along with the respective calorie content. Eat your proteins, fruits, and vegetables!

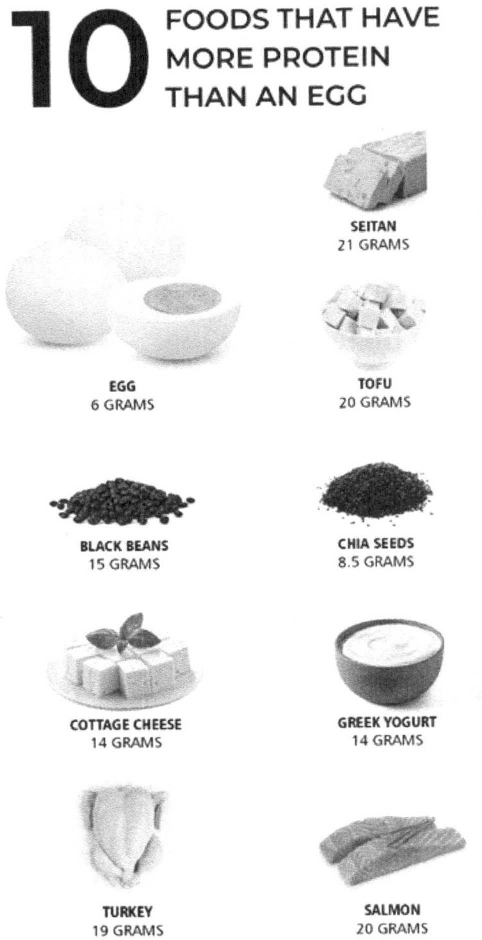
10 FOODS THAT HAVE MORE PROTEIN THAN AN EGG
SEITAN
21 GRAMS
EGG
6 GRAMS
TOFU
20 GRAMS
BLACK BEANS
15 GRAMS
CHIA SEEDS
8.5 GRAMS
COTTAGE CHEESE
14 GRAMS
GREEK YOGURT
14 GRAMS
TURKEY
19 GRAMS
SALMON
20 GRAMS

Protein sources can be plant-based, such as soy beans, nuts, seeds, and legumes, or animal-based, like meat or dairy. The following image is a list of healthy animal and plant-based proteins, along with their respective protein content.

ANIMAL VS PLANT PROTEINS

Animal Proteins: Depending on their source, proteins can be plant-based or animal-based. Animal-based proteins include fish, chicken, beef, turkey, eggs, etc. Plant-based proteins can be found in soy, fruits, beets, nuts, and seeds.

Here are some differences between these two proteins:

COMPLETE VS. INCOMPLETE PROTEIN

Animal proteins, particularly meat, poultry, fish, eggs, and dairy, contain all nine essential amino acids and are a good source of complete protein.

Many plant-based foods, like grains, nuts, and seeds, may lack one or more of these essential amino acids. Some other plant-based sources, like soy protein and soy derivatives, could be complete proteins, but many others are incomplete. Please refer to the next section for complete soy derivative products.

Health Benefits:

According to the research, plant-based proteins are lower in saturated fat and cholesterol and higher in fiber, vitamins, and minerals, which may reduce the risk of chronic diseases like heart disease, diabetes, and some cancers. A diet high in fiber could promote gut health and help with weight loss.

Animal proteins also while containing all essential amino acids, animal protein sources can be higher in saturated fat and cholesterol. Consumption of processed or unprocessed red meat has been associated with an increased risk of mortality by 13%, as per some research studies, and increases the risk of heart disease. Lean meats and fish can help with weight loss and reduce cardiovascular risk factors.

Muscle Building:

While animal proteins were once considered superior for building muscle mass, new research suggests that plant-based proteins, like those found in nuts and beans, can be just as effective. However, studies on the effect of protein source on lean mass and muscle strength are still ongoing.

On plant plant-based diet, you have to make sure you add enough zinc, B12, calcium, and Vitamin D. To get the nutrition you need on a plant-based diet, eat fortified cereals, whole grains, and beans for zinc. You might have to take B12 supplements or add nutritional yeast to a plant-based diet to get B12. Lots of green leafy vegetables for calcium.

HEALTHY ANIMAL-BASED PROTEINS:

Lean meats usually have low fat content. They refer to cuts of meat, such as chicken, turkey, pork, or beef, that have been trimmed of visible fat. Lean meats usually contain less than 10 grams of total fat, 4-5 grams or less saturated fat, and less than 95 milligrams of cholesterol per 100 grams. Skinless chicken, Turkey breast, pork cuts like tenderloin and sirloin, and lean ground beef are good examples of lean meats and are usually considered healthy meats.

- **Poultry:** Skinless Chicken and Turkey, Lean Ground Turkey or Chicken, Chicken Tenderloin, Chicken Thigh. Chicken thigh is a good source of protein, iron, and B vitamins, especially when skinless. Poultry is a good source of vitamin B12.
- **Beef:** leaner cuts like top sirloin, round steaks (eye round, top round, and bottom round), and chuck shoulder are generally lower in fat and higher in protein, making them a good choice for a balanced diet.
- Beef is an excellent source of iron and zinc.
- **Pork:** Pork tenderloin, loin chops, and center loin are lean cuts. Bacon and other fatty cuts are very high in artery-clogging saturated fat and cholesterol, and are not for everyday eating.
- **Fish and Seafood:** Most fish and seafood are naturally lean, including white-fleshed fish like cod, tilapia, and mahi-mahi, as well as shrimp. Other healthy options like salmon, sardines, oysters, and trout are also a good source of Omega-3 Fatty acids.
- **Other Lean Options:** Venison.

HOW TO CHOOSE HEALTHY, LEAN MEATS:

- **Read the label:** Choose beef or pork labeled 90% lean or higher.
- **Trim visible fat:** Remove excess fat from the meat before cooking.
- **Choose skinless poultry:** Opt for skinless chicken or turkey to reduce saturated fat.

SOY PROTEIN:

Vegan and vegetarian people often struggle with healthy protein sources. Soy protein could be a good option for them. Soy protein is found in a variety of food derivatives of Soy Beans, such as tofu, tempeh, edamame, soy milk, and miso. Soy protein concentrate, soy isolates, and soy flour are used in various protein meal replacements and processed foods.

Let's understand soy products in detail. It can help us add variety to the food. All these products are easily available at the grocery stores.

Unfermented Soy products:

- **Tofu:** A soft, firm, or hard consistency, white, custard-like product made from coagulated soy milk.
- **Edamame:** Young, immature soybeans in their pods, eaten raw or steamed
- **Soy Milk:** A liquid made from soybeans

- **Soybeans:** The whole bean itself, which can be eaten dry, roasted, or cooked.
- **Soy nuts:** Roasted soybeans, offering a crunchy and flavorful snack option.

Fermented Soy Products:

- **Tempeh:** A fermented soybean patty, often containing other grains to enhance its protein content.
- **Miso:** A fermented soybean paste used as a seasoning in various dishes, particularly in Japanese cuisine.
- **Natto:** A fermented soybean dish, also known as fermented soybeans, with a sticky, slightly slimy texture.

Processed Soy Products:

Soy Protein Concentrate:

A protein-rich ingredient used in various food products, often found in plant-based meat alternatives.

Soy Flour:

A ground product made from soybeans, used in baking and various other food applications.

Soy Protein Isolate:

A highly concentrated soy protein, often used in supplements and certain processed foods.

Nuts, seeds, whole grains, Greek yogurt, legumes, and meal replacements could be an alternative source of protein.

Please refer to the chart below for the protein content of animal and plant proteins:

Nutritional Food Chart (Animal-Based & Dairy Sources)

Category	Food	Typical Portion	Protein (g)	Calories
Fish & Seafood	Sardines (canned)	1 small can	25	220
	Salmon	3 oz	22	130
	Tuna	3 oz	22	100
	Rainbow trout	3 oz	20	145
	Shrimp	3 oz	20	100
	Scallops	3 oz	14	75
Meat	Lean beef (round)	3 oz	25	140
	Steak (moderate cut)	3 oz	23	260
	Extra-lean ground beef	3 oz	22	230
	Pork tenderloin	3 oz	24	140
	Pork loin	3 oz	24	180
Poultry	Chicken breast (skinless)	3 oz	18	100
	Chicken thigh (skinless)	1 thigh	14	110
	Turkey breast (skinless)	3 oz	25	115
	Deli turkey	1 slice	4	25
Eggs	Whole egg	1 large	6	75
	Egg white	1 large	4	15
Dairy	Greek yogurt (low-fat)	1 cup	23	170
	Yogurt (low-fat)	1 cup	13	150
	Cottage cheese (low-fat)	½ cup	12	100
	Skim milk	1 cup	8	90

Nutritional Food Chart (Plant-Based Sources)

Category	Food	Typical Portion	Protein (g)	Calories
Plant Proteins	Tempeh	3 oz	15	165
	Tofu (firm)	3 oz	12	110
	Tofu (soft)	3 oz	4	50
Legumes	Lentils (cooked)	½ cup	9	100
	Black beans	½ cup	8	115
	Chickpeas	½ cup	7	135
	Kidney beans	½ cup	8	110
	Edamame	½ cup	9	95
Nuts & Seeds	Almonds	¼ cup	6	170
	Peanuts	¼ cup	7	165
	Pumpkin seeds	¼ cup	9	160
	Chia seeds	2 Tbsp	5	140
	Peanut butter	1 Tbsp	7	190
Grains	Quinoa (cooked)	1 cup	8	225
	Oatmeal (cooked)	1 cup	11	300
	Whole-wheat pasta	1 cup	8	180
	Whole-grain bread	1 slice	3	85

4.3 Carbohydrates

Carbohydrates are not just the first fuel tank of our body, but also the primary source of energy. They are the main energy source for our body, fueling essential functions like brain activity, muscle movement, and nerve function. Carbohydrates are classified into simple or complex. Depending on the structure, they are also classified as monosaccharides, disaccharides, oligosaccharides, or polysaccharides.

Carbohydrates are classified as sugars, fibers, and starches. Sugar is the simplest form of carbohydrate, while starches or fiber are complex forms. The body's primary source of energy, fueling essential functions like brain activity, muscle movement, and nerve function. Fiber, a crucial component of carbohydrates, aids digestion and helps regulate blood cholesterol, providing a sense of reassurance about the health benefits of carbohydrates. The body stores extra carbohydrates as glycogen in muscles and the liver for later use. Simple carbohydrates are quickly digested and absorbed, causing a rapid rise in blood sugar, while complex carbohydrates are digested more slowly and provide sustained energy. While both simple and complex carbs are needed in the diet, it is often advised to add more complex carbs to the diet for weight management.

The following chart shows a list of simple and complex carbs. You are well advised to choose more complex carbs in your diet.

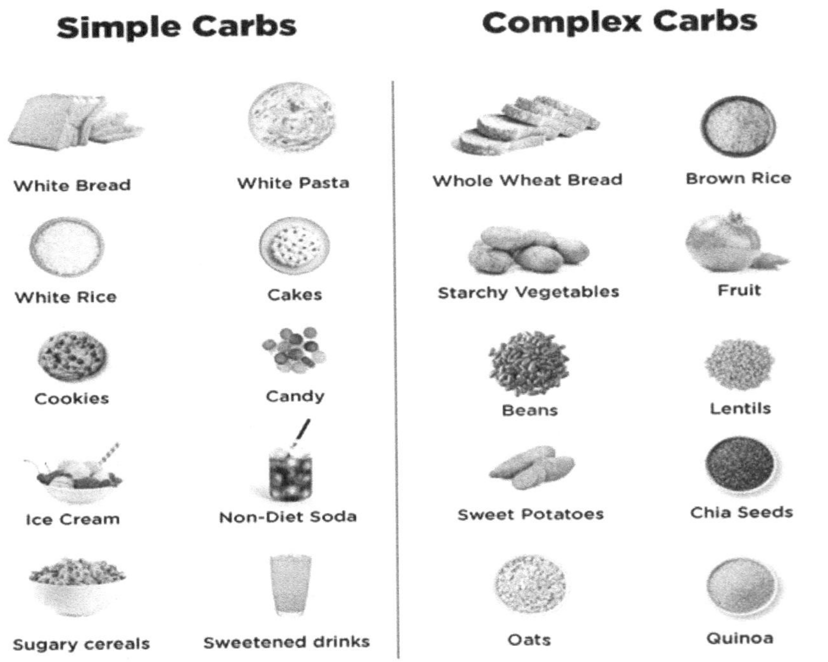

Carbohydrates are classified into Sugars, starches, and fibers. Let's go over this individually.

Sugars

Sugars are a type of simple carbohydrate. Your body breaks down and absorbs simple carbohydrates quickly, raising blood sugar levels quickly, but levels fall quickly as well, giving a feeling of fatigue and tiredness. All the extra sugar and simple carbs are converted into fats and stored in the body for later usage.

There are two types of sugars:

- Naturally occurring sugars, like those found in milk and fresh fruits.
- Added sugars, like those found in sweets, canned fruit, juice, and soda. Sweets include things like cookies, candy bars, and ice cream.

Sugar goes by many names. On food labels, you may see sugar listed as:

- Agave nectar.
- Cane syrup or corn syrup.
- Dextrose, fructose, or sucrose.
- Honey.
- Molasses.
- Sugar.

Limiting sugar is essential to keep your blood sugar levels in the healthy range.

Sugary foods and drinks are often higher in calories, which can contribute to weight gain.

Limit refined foods containing added sugar, like white flour, desserts, candy, juices, fruit drinks, soda pop, and sweetened beverages.

The sugar intake as recommended by American Heart Association:

- Women: ≤ 25 g/day (6 tsp)
- Men: ≤ 36 g/day (9 tsp)

- Children (2-18): ≤ 25 g/day (6 tsp)
- Children < 2: Avoid added sugar

Starches

Starches are complex carbohydrates that also give your body vitamins and minerals (micronutrients). It takes your body longer to break down complex carbohydrates. As a result, starches help regulate sugars and also help you stay full for long hours.

You can find starchy carbohydrates in:

- Beans and legumes, like black beans, chickpeas, lentils, lima beans, and kidney beans.
- Fruits, like apples, berries, and melons.
- Whole-grain products, like brown rice, oatmeal, and whole-wheat bread and pasta.
- Vegetables, like corn, peas, and potatoes.

Fiber

Fiber is a complex healthy carbohydrate with lots of health benefits. Fibers are of two types: soluble and insoluble. Your body can't break down fiber well, but soluble fiber can dissolve in water, whereas insoluble fiber can't. Fiber helps form the bulk of stool in the intestine, stimulates and aids digestion, prevents constipation, promotes gut health, and the growth of healthy bacteria.

Studies show that a high-fiber diet can help reduce cholesterol, regulate sugar, and keep people full for long hours.

Fruits, vegetables, nuts, grains, and psyllium are examples of soluble fiber, while Corn is an example of insoluble fiber.

Experts recommend that adults consume 25 to 30 grams (g) of fiber every day. Most people get half that amount.

High-fiber foods include:

- Beans and legumes, like black beans, chickpeas, lentils, lima beans, peanuts, and pinto beans.
- Fruits, especially those with edible skins (apples and peaches) or seeds (berries).
- Nuts and seeds, including almonds, walnuts, pumpkin seeds, and sunflower seeds.
- Whole-grain products, like brown rice, oatmeal, quinoa, cereal, and whole-wheat bread and pasta.
- Vegetables, like corn, broccoli, brussels sprouts, and squash.

On average, 45% to 65% of your calories could be coming from carbohydrates. So, if someone is on a 2000-calorie diet, close to 900 to 1300 calories could be coming from carbohydrates. Each molecule of carbohydrate gives 4.5 calories.

What are complex carbs?

Complex carbohydrates are the ones that have more fiber and polysaccharides.

What is the difference between net carbs and total carbs?

Total carb is the carb plus fiber. When you take the fiber out, that is called carbs. Understanding this difference can help you make informed choices when reading nutrition labels. Always look at labeled food with more fiber. Less net carbs are healthy.

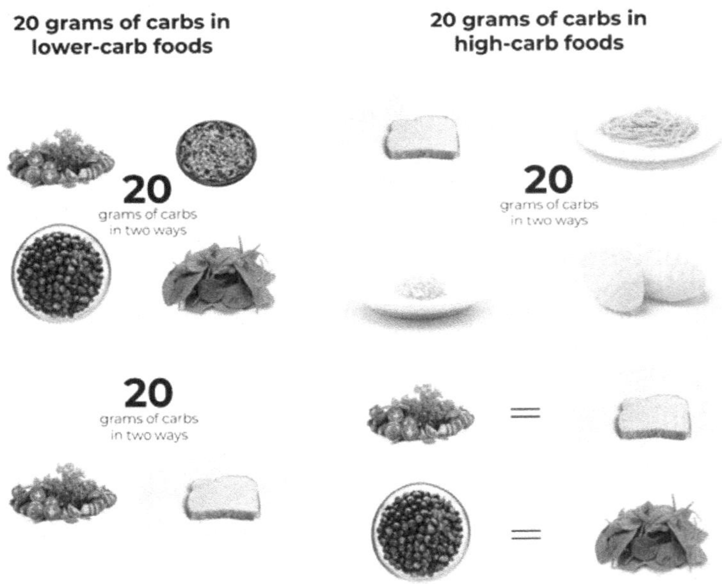

Choose your carbs carefully:

10 Healthiest Carbs

1. Quinoa
2. Buckwheat
3. Oat meal
4. Beans
5. Fruits and vegetables
6. Sweet potatoes
7. Lentils
8. Sorghum
9. Millets
10. Brown rice

4.4 Fats

Fat molecules are primarily made of carbon and hydrogen atoms in cholesterol, phospholipids, and triglycerides. Fats are viewed as unhealthy, but they are needed for multiple metabolic functions and are also an important part of the human diet. Fats can be saturated, unsaturated, trans unsaturated, or polyunsaturated. Omega fats are generally saturated. Trans fats are considered unhealthy, whereas monosaturated and polysaturated fatty acids are considered healthier and a better source for our body.

As per general guidelines, the fat intake should be

limited to less than 10% of your calories consumed per day. So, if you are on a 1500-calorie diet, less than 150 calories should be coming from fats. One fat molecule gives 9 calories. So, fat intake should be less than 20 g a day.

GOOD FATS Use These	**BAD FATS** Loose These
Salmon	Crackers
Eggs	French Fries
Organic Nut Oils	Hydrogenated Oils
Olive Oil	Pastries
Avocados	Margarine
Coconut Oil	Doughnuts
Flaxseed	Processed Meats
Raw Nuts	Cookies
Leafy Green Vegetables	Canola Oil
Organic Butter	

4.5 Fiber

Fibers are also covered in the carbohydrate section. Another important component of diet is fiber. Fiber can either be water soluble or water insoluble.

Water-soluble fiber is found inside plants. It swells up when it comes in contact with water.

On average, men need 35 g of fiber in their diet, and women need 28 g daily.

Here are some excellent sources of fiber:

- **Vegetables:** Broccoli, Brussels sprouts, carrots, cauliflower, celery, cucumbers, green beans, peas, potatoes (with skin), and spinach.
- **Fruits:** Apples, berries (strawberries, blueberries, and raspberries), bananas, grapes, oranges, pears, and raisins.
- **Legumes:** Beans, kidney, black peas, pinto, chickpeas, lentils, peas.
- **Nuts and Seeds:** Almonds, chia seeds, flaxseeds, oatmeal, pistachios, and walnuts.
- **Other Sources:** Whole-grain breads, cereals, popcorn, and granola.

100-calorie snacks

25 HEALTHY 100 CALORIE SNACK LIST

Nuts & Seeds

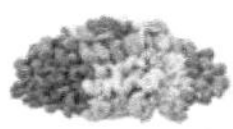

- 14 almonds
- 12 cashews
- 10 walnut halves
- 2 tbsp sunflower seeds
- 1 tbsp peanut butter on celery
- 1 tbsp chia seeds in water
- 1.5 tbsp pumpkin seeds

Dairy & Alternatives

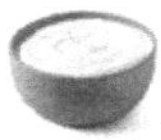

- ½ cup low-fat Greek yogurt
- 1 string cheese
- ¾ cup skim milk
- 1¼ cup cottage cheese
- ½ cup unsweetened soy milk
- 1 oz feta cheese with cucumber slices
- 1 oz mozzarella cheese

Fruits (Fresh or Dried)

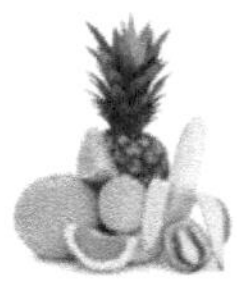

- 1 medium apple
- 1 small banana
- 1 cup blueberries
- 1 cup strawberries
- ½ mango
- 1 cup watermelon
- ½ cup grapes
- 2 dried apricots + 5 almonds
- ½ small avocado with lime and chilli

Whole Grains

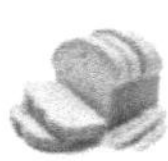

- 1 slice whole-grain bread
- ½ whole wheat English muffin
- 2 tbsp oatmeal (dry) with cinnamon
- ½ granola bar (check label)
- 1 mini corn tortilla + 1 tsp guacamole
- 3 plain rice cakes
- 1 mini whole wheat pita

Vegetables

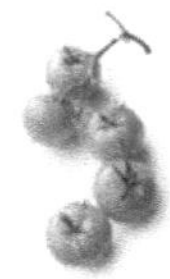

- 1 cup baby carrots with 1 tbsp hummus
- 1 cucumber with lemon and chilli powder
- 1 bell pepper sliced with 2 tbsp salsa
- 1 cup cherry tomatoes + 1 string cheese
- 2 cups air-popped popcorn
- 1 cup edamame (steamed, unsalted)
- 1 small sweet potato, baked
- 1 cup roasted zucchini or eggplant

Protein-Packed Snacks

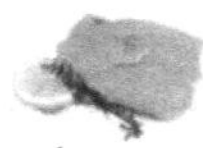

- 1 hard-boiled egg
- 2 egg whites scrambled with spinach
- 1 oz turkey breast rolled with lettuce
- ½ can tuna (in water)
- 1 oz grilled chicken breast
- 1 slice smoked salmon on cucumber
- 2 tbsp hummus with raw veggies
- 2 tbsp cottage cheese with cherry tomatoes
- 2 falafel balls (small baked)

Light Treats

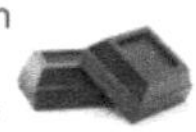

- 1 small square dark chocolate
- 1 frozen banana slice dipped in chocolate
- 1 mini frozen Greek yogurt bar
- 1 tbsp cocoa powder in almond milk
- 1 tbsp mini chocolate chips + berries
- 2 squares dark chocolate + green tea

Drinks & Smooth Options

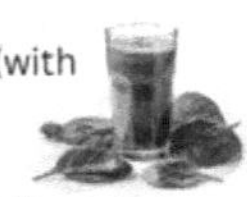

- 1 cup almond milk smoothie (with spinach/berries)
- ½ protein shake (low sugar)
- 1 cup unsweetened iced tea + lemon
- 1 small fruit + veggie juice (unsweetened)
- 1 coconut water box (small)
- 1 glass lemon-cucumber detox water

4.6 MY HEALTHY PLATE

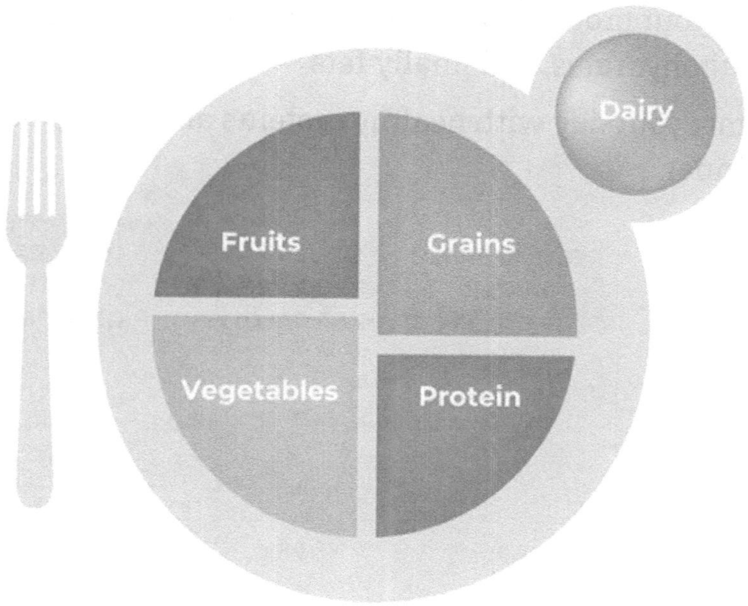

The best way to put all proteins, carbs, and fats into a plate is to use my healthy plate. In other words, each 1/4th part of your plate must contain proteins, fruits, grains, and vegetables.

Now, as you have a list of healthy carbohydrates, grains, proteins, and fats, please pick your food carefully and fill your plate with nutrition.

Irrespective of the kind of diet plan you wish to follow, here are some basic rules that could apply to dieting:

- 20 to 25 g of protein in every meal
- 10 to 15 g of protein in each snack

- More complex carbohydrates like quinoa, whole-grain flour, and brown rice instead of simple carbs
- Eat your proteins, vegetables, and fruits first, followed by carbohydrates, and finally fats
- Start your day with healthy proteins and keep it light on dinner.

	RECOMMENDED RANGES (% OF CALORIES)	LOWER CARB HIGHER PROTEIN (% OF CALORIES)	LOWER CARB & FAT HIGHER PROTIEN
CARBS	45-65%	45%	45%
PROTEINS	10-35%	25%	30%
FAT	20-35%	30%	25%

4.7 Alcohol (ETOH) and Obesity

What is alcohol exactly? We all know that it is fermented sugar coming from grape juice or grains when yeast/ bacteria are introduced to liquid containing sugar and microorganisms convert sugars into ethanol and carbon dioxide. While the sugar in fruits and grains is converted to alcohol and carbon dioxide during fermentation, some drinks retain residual sugar or have sugar added for flavoring or to increase alcohol content. Additionally, many alcoholic beverages are mixed with sugary drinks like soda, juice, or liqueurs, which significantly increase the sugar content.

Here is the sugar content of various alcoholic beverages:

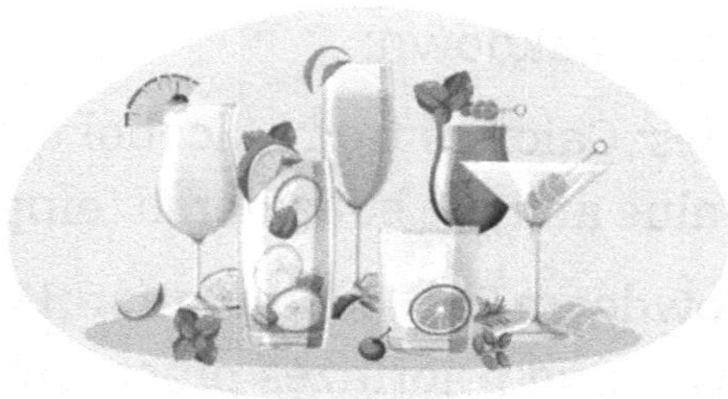

Type of alcohol	Serving size	Amount of carbs (grams)
BEER (REGULAR)	12 oz (355 ml)	12-15
WINE (RED)	5 oz (150 ml)	3-4
WINE (WHITE)	5 oz (150 ml)	3-4
VODKA	1.5 oz (45 ml)	0
RUM	1.5 oz (45 ml)	0
GIN	1.5 oz (45 ml)	0
WHISKEY	1.5 oz (45 ml)	0-0.5
MARGARITA	4 oz (120 ml)	10-15
MOJITO	6 oz (180 ml)	25-30
LONG ISLAND ICED TEA	8 oz (240 ml)	33-40

Alcohol can contribute to weight gain through various mechanisms, including providing empty calories, slowing down metabolism, and increasing appetite and abdominal fat. The body recognizes alcohol as a toxin and prioritizes its elimination through metabolism rather than other metabolic functions like fat burning, leading to weight gain.

Here's a detailed breakdown:

- **Empty Calories:** Calories from Alcohol carry little or no nutritional value and are considered "empty calories"
- **Metabolic Slowdown/fat accumulation:** Body recognizes alcohol as toxin and prioritizes processing alcohol over other metabolic processes which can lead to other calories being stored as fat. Increased fat around belly is called beer belly
- **Increased Appetite:** Alcohol can stimulate appetite and increase cravings for high-calorie foods, especially salty and fatty foods, leading to overeating and weight gain
- **Disrupted Sleep:** Alcohol can disrupt sleep patterns, leading to poor quality of sleep. Sleep deprivation is linked to increased appetite and cravings, making it harder to lose weight.

The body can't store alcohol as an energy source for later usage.

Factors affecting ETOH metabolism:

While talking about alcohol we also have to keep in mind how alcohol is broken down in the body. 90 to 98% of alcohol is metabolized in the liver with the help of enzyme called ADH converted into acetaldehyde(toxic substance) than in broken down into at Acetate (less toxic substance) the help of aldehyde dehydrogenase (ALDH) finally into carbon monoxide and water and eliminated from the body. As acetaldehyde is a toxic substance its conversion to acetate with the help of aldehyde dehydrogenase is very crucial step.

The activity of ALDH varies among people primarily due to genetic variations in the ALDH2 gene. This is particularly evident in populations of East Asian descent, leading to flushing and more side effects from alcohol consumption.

Drinking alcohol on an empty stomach leads to faster absorption of alcohol into the bloodstream, resulting in quicker intoxication and potentially higher blood alcohol content (BAC).

Sugar content and the kind of ETOH consumed are other important aspects. Please refer to the chart given above for the sugar content of individual drinks.

In conclusion, while alcohol can contribute to weight gain, the extent of its impact depends on various factors, including the amount and type of alcohol consumed, individual metabolism, and overall lifestyle. While cutting down on alcohol can have a strong impact on weight management, using alcohol in moderation can mitigate some side effects from alcohol consumption.

4.8 MEDITERRANEAN DIET

"Mediterranean diet" is a generic term based on the traditional eating habits in the countries bordering the Mediterranean Sea.

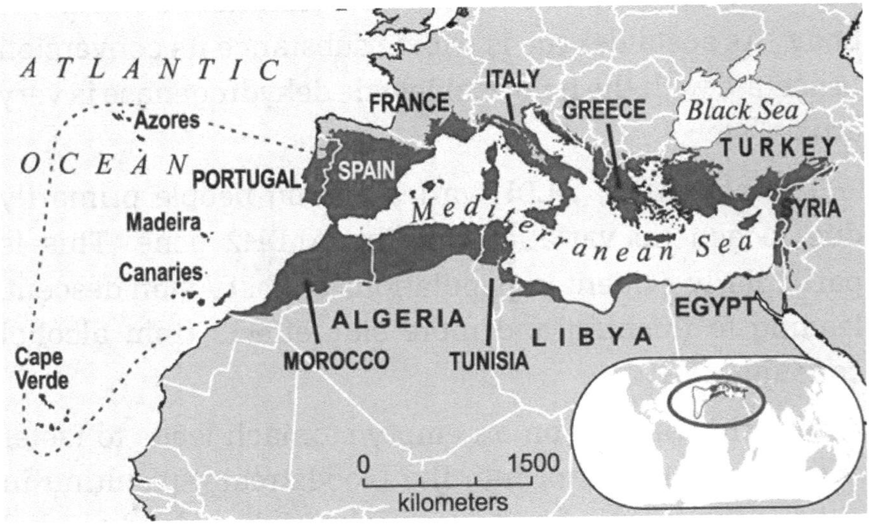

At least 16 countries share their border with the Mediterranean Sea. All of them vary in culture, ethnic background, religion, economy, geography, and agricultural produce. However, there are some common factors. All of them include:

- Plenty of fruits, vegetables, bread and other grains, potatoes, beans, nuts, and seeds
- Olive oil as a primary fat source
- Dairy products, eggs, fish, and poultry in low to moderate amounts
- Fish and poultry are more common than red meat
- Minimally processed, plant-based, low sugar

- Fruit is a dessert instead of sweets
- Wine may be consumed in low to moderate amounts, usually with a meal.

The Mediterranean diet is widely recognized as one of the healthiest eating patterns globally, associated with numerous health benefits such as lower blood pressure, reduced risk of heart disease, and better blood sugar control. Despite its popularity, many individuals are not fully aware of its specific characteristics. While most people associate the diet with ingredients like olive oil, fish, fruits, and vegetables, its true essence is more intricate.

Unlike MyPlate in the US, which outlines what foods to include in each meal, the Mediterranean Diet emphasizes a broader approach, focusing on the frequency of food consumption, i.e., daily, weekly, and monthly. Ultimately, it promotes a lifestyle choice rather than merely a temporary dietary plan.

Foods that should be eaten:

Daily: Whole grains, fruits, vegetables, beans, nuts, olive oil (the main fat source), and dairy (yogurt and cheese).

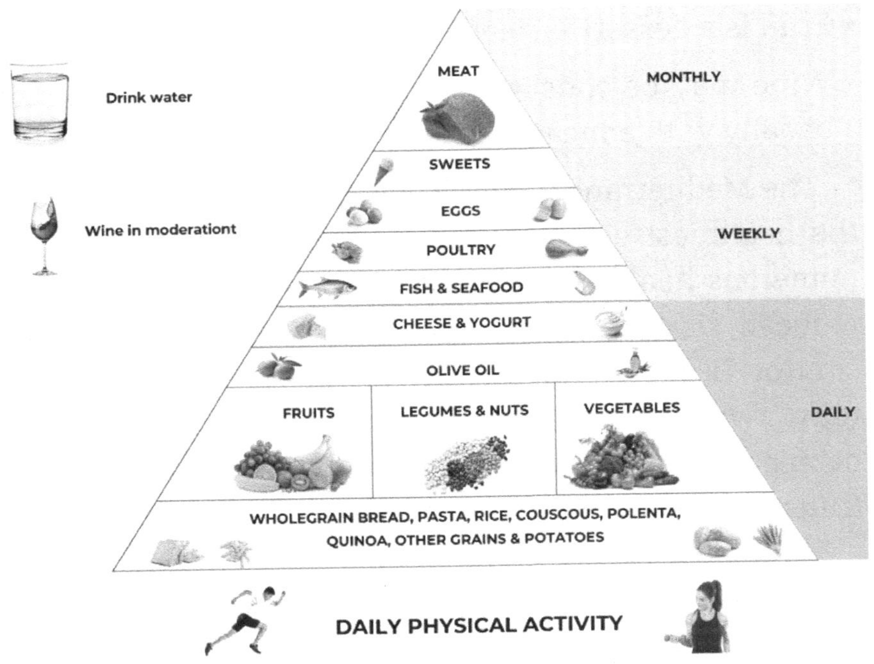

Weekly: Fish and poultry. Sweets in moderation.

Dessert: A piece of fruit or fruit salad.

Monthly: Sweets with higher sugar content are reserved for special occasions.

Practical Aspects

Portion control and moderation are important parts of the Mediterranean diet. Many Italians enjoy their meals slowly and stop eating when they feel full. Meals usually come in smaller portions. It is uncommon to have more than one or two glasses of wine with a meal.

You might not find certain items, like salad dressing, in large grocery stores. If you love ranch dressing, you will need to adjust when ordering a salad here. Salads are typically dressed only with olive oil and balsamic vinegar, which may take some getting used to.

Adopting the Mediterranean style of diet completely may not be practical in the United States, but one can certainly incorporate some of the diet items into daily life.

ABC technique:

A - Awareness → B - Behavior → C - Change

A - Awareness: What Are You Really Eating?

"To notice is the beginning of transformation."

Here you learn how different foods affect you body, weight, energy, and health. Understanding the role of calories, carbohydrates, and fats is essential for making informed choices about nutrition and energy balance. Calories in versus calories out is a key principle, while the quality of carbohydrates is more important than simply counting grams - whole grains and fiber-rich carbs are preferable. Fats shouldn't be feared, but it's best to avoid trans fats and instead focus on healthy unsaturated fats like those found in avocados, nuts, and olive oil. Macronutrients such as proteins support muscle repair, satiety, and metabolism; carbohydrates provide quick energy and should be sourced from whole foods; fats are vital for hormone production and brain health. Fiber, often overlooked, helps slow digestion, balance blood sugar, and support gut health.

Alcohol can contribute to weight gain through empty

calories, disrupted metabolism, and increased cravings. A balanced approach to nutrition, such as following the Mediterranean Diet, emphasizes anti-inflammatory benefits and heart health, with a healthy plate being ideally divided into half vegetables and fruits, one-quarter protein, and one-quarter grains, favoring overall well-being over fad diets.

Reflections:

- What food or nutrient do I fear, and where did that belief come from?

- How balanced is my plate at most meals?

- How does alcohol show up in my lifestyle - and how does it affect my food choices?

B - Behavior: Small Shifts in How You Eat

"Nutrition habits are built meal by meal, not by perfection."

Now translate this knowledge into small, intentional dietary habits they can sustain over time. Being mindful of portion sizes - such as filling half your plate with vegetables, using your palm to gauge protein, and your fist for starch - can foster balanced meals without the need for constant calorie counting. Learning to read nutrition labels helps you spot added sugars, trans fats, and excess sodium, making it easier to swap soda for sparkling water or white bread for whole grain alternatives. Including protein with every meal not only boosts satiety but also supports a healthy metabolism, while naturally increasing fiber intake through beans, lentils, flaxseeds, vegetables, and fruits can enhance digestion and gut health.

Mindful drinking, for instance by "budgeting" alcohol to just one or two drinks per week and avoiding drinking alone, supports healthier choices overall. Embracing a Mediterranean-style approach - prioritizing olive oil, herbs, fish, nuts, legumes, whole grains, and more plant-based meals - offers a simple yet powerful foundation for sustained well-being.

Reflections:

- What's one eating habit I'd like to adjust - not restrict?

- How can I add more fiber or protein to my next meal?

- What does a "Mediterranean-style" meal look like for me?

C - Change: Building a Nourishing Lifestyle

"Food isn't just fuel - it's culture, connection, and healing."

Here you move from temporary "dieting" to a sustainable way of eating aligned with you health and identity.

Moving from restriction to nourishment means reframing your mindset from thinking "I can't have this" to intentionally choosing foods that serve you and your well-being. It involves designing your food environment - arranging your home, preparing your grocery lists, and planning your schedule - to set yourself up for success without unnecessary stress. Planning meals becomes a tool for support rather than obsession: batch cooking, crafting simple weekly plans, and allowing for flexibility ensure that nourishment is both achievable and enjoyable. Setting boundaries with alcohol, such as adopting the identity of someone who drinks less and feels better, can further reinforce these positive shifts. Ultimately, embracing the new dietary lifestyle in your own way - through joyful eating, home-cooked meals, and social gatherings that prioritize health - lays a strong foundation for sustained, vibrant living.

Reflections:

• What does "eating well" mean to me - emotionally and physically?

• What food choices help me feel most energized and balanced?

• What's one new food habit that feels sustainable and aligned with who I want to be?

Chapter : 5

Physical Activity

"Lack of activity destroys the good condition of every human being, while movement and methodical physical exercise save it and preserve it."

-Plato

THE MOVEMENT QUESTION

This chapter is about making physical activity simple, realistic, and something you can actually enjoy. Small, consistent steps can build strength, energy, and confidence over time.

5.1 Sitting and watching our health decline

Do you know that the average American sits for 7 to 8 hours? This is the primary reason why people plateau and are unable to lose weight, because they have a sedentary job. Sitting for long hours affects our muscles.

Here are some facts about sitting, though they are statements; each statement has clinical research behind it.

Since your core muscles are less active in a sitting position, they weaken. The hip flexor gets shortened and tight. It decreases the blood flow to the legs, causing a circulation problem. It causes significant weakening of our muscles.

There are some shocking facts about sitting. There is research behind each of the following statements.

How does sitting
impact my posture?

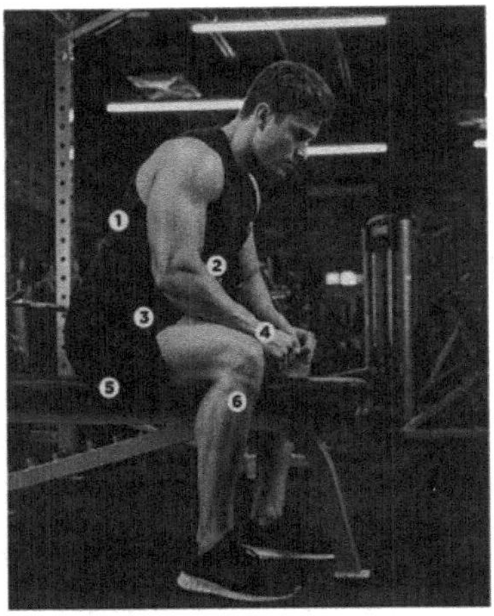

1 **Redistribution of weight to lower back**
Stress on the lower back, higher intradiscal pressure, impinged nerve roots

2 **Core muscles are less active**
Muscles weaken, unable to support the body

3 **Hip flexor shorten & tighten**
Pull on the pelvis, causing anterior tilt and strain in the lower back

4 **Hamstrings shorten & tighten**
Pull on the pelvis, flattening the lower back

5 **Glute muscles disengage**
Muscles weaken and become soft/unde-fined

6 **Decreased blood flow to legs**
Circulation and nerve problems

Multiple studies suggest

- Sitting for more than 8hours/day can increase the risk of developing heart disease
- Your body's ability to process insulin decreases by sitting for long hours on one day. This increases the risk of diabetes
- When you are sitting, it affects your body functioning because of decreased blood flow to the brain
- An hour of intense workout doesn't compensate for 7 hours of sitting during the day
- When you are sitting for longer hours, it affects your back muscles.

Actionable Plan

First and foremost, it is important to increase our awareness while sitting for long hours. Breaking this habit is the first step. We all have office jobs that require us to sit and focus on a task. So, getting up every hour to stretch or even for a small walk becomes crucial.

Increasing your non-exercise activities, like parking your car far away from the workplace, going for a walk during lunch break, or having a standing desk at the job, can be a few simple practices that prevent us from sitting for long hours.

5.2 Why is it important to exercise?

According to a survey, not taking care of the body and not exercising was one of the major regrets in elderly age.

"To know the road ahead, ask those who are coming back."

Exercise has unlimited benefits!

During exercise, our muscle cells utilize glucose as their primary energy source. These muscle cells experience a surge in their glucose demand. This prompts the pancreas to decrease the release of insulin, a hormone crucial for glucose regulation. Over time, it enhances insulin sensitivity, effectively combating insulin resistance.

Moreover, the benefits of exercise extend beyond just metabolic health. When we exercise, our heart rate elevates, pumping blood more forcefully through our arteries. This surge in blood circulation is especially beneficial for the brain, where enhanced blood flow delivers vital oxygen and nutrients. They can profoundly increase concentration, sharpen memory, and enhance cognitive abilities, making even simple tasks feel more manageable and enjoyable.

In addition to its physiological benefits, exercise acts as a powerful antidote to the stresses of daily life. Each workout produces a surge of endorphins, often referred to as feel-good hormones, that flow through the body, inducing a sense of euphoria and relaxation.

Embracing a routine of physical activity not only strengthens our bodies but also enriches our mental state, cultivating resilience, joy, and a profound sense of well-being. By weaving exercise into the fabric of our daily lives, we transform our physical health. We paint a vibrant, holistic portrait of optimal living.

5.3 How to start?

The night before going to bed, many of us feel highly motivated to start exercising the next day. However, when the alarm goes off, that motivation often fades away. Mel Robbins, a motivational speaker, once said, "Motivation is garbage!" It tends to vanish when we need it the most. So, how can we actually begin exercising?

First, avoid setting yourself a tough task, especially for the morning. Getting out of bed and starting a daily chore is already something our brains naturally resist. If you follow that with a demanding task, like running on a treadmill, it increases the chances you will want to give up entirely.

Instead, let us use the SMART goal framework to set simple objectives. Begin with something manageable, like walking for just 10 minutes. You can also engage in activities that you truly enjoy, such as dancing, listening to music, yoga, or stretching.

To successfully change your lifestyle, it is important to start with something you enjoy. Research suggests that it takes 21 days to transform a lifestyle, and about 6 months for that change to become a habit.

Having an exercise partner can prove beneficial. So, consider working out with someone you know, either your spouse or a friend. While choosing a workout partner, it would be great if that person's overall health and lifestyle match yours. This would ensure setting similar fitness goals and adhering to them.

Prepare your exercise clothes the night before to make it easier to get started. Invest in some nice workout clothes that you look forward to wearing. Begin with simple exercises and gradually increase the intensity as you progress.

5.4 Seated Work-Outs

This section is specifically devoted to those people who have limited physical activity due to any medical condition, or even people who have a job that requires long hours of sitting.

It is specifically beneficial for people whose physical activities are limited. Here are some simple exercises that you can perform while sitting in a chair. Of course, it is advisable that you stand, stretch, or walk around at least once every hour. This will not only regulate your blood circulation but also allow your back and leg muscles to relax.

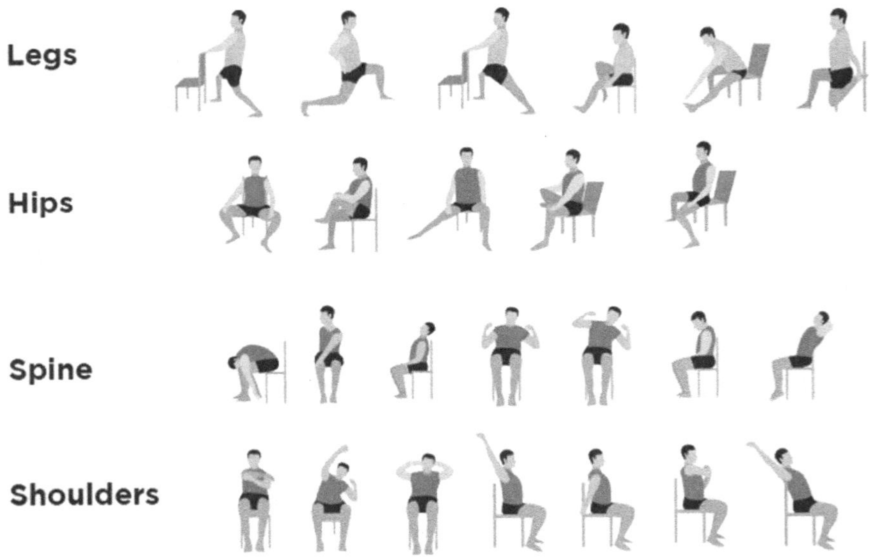

5.5 Cardio and Core Exercises

Do you know that you have to run for 36 minutes at a speed of 3-5 miles per hour to burn the calories consumed from having a cookie and 46 minutes at the same speed to burn the calories from 1 slice of pizza. It takes only a minute or 2 to have these foods.

Running is an exercise that increases your heart rate. The maximum heart rate that you can achieve is your age multiplied by 0.7 and subtracted from 220. This is why you should push yourself as much as possible while exercising. Do not limit yourself to gentle exercise like walking if you are in your 30s or 40s. Even if you are in your 50s or 60s and engage in brisk walking as a form of exercise, try walking as fast as you can with exaggerated side movements of both hands. It should be no less than at least 40 minutes to call it a cardio exercise. You may listen to fast-paced music on the go to get in the rhythm. You do not need a partner for this exercise. There is no point chatting while you are brisk walking because it will only decrease your speed and focus.

We often hear people complaining about not being able to lose weight despite walking miles and miles. Fat loss needs high-intensity exercise. Walking is a low-intensity workout. Walking is good to relieve stress, but it is not good enough to burn the fat that hangs around your waist.

Fat-burning hormones need higher-intensity workouts, like running, cycling, or swimming. Though a large percentage of calories are burned, the total amount of fat burned is negligible while walking. Added to this is that the moment you stop walking, the metabolism is back to baseline, and you stop burning calories. To really burn stubborn fat, you need to walk 2 to 5 hours close or 10,000 to 20,000 steps, daily. However, that would seem impractical to most of us.

So, what is the best way to do the exercise that can really burn that stubborn fat? The answer to this is doing a high-intensity workout. Instead of engaging in a monotonous exercise for long hours, it is better to perform high-intensity workouts.

Exercise as a Marker of Fitness:

To understand exercise as a marker of fitness, let us go over the concept of VO2. VO2 (max oxygen consumption) is the highest rate at which a person can use oxygen during intense exercise.

VO2 max is a key indicator of cardiovascular fitness and aerobic endurance. A higher VO2 max indicates that a person can use oxygen more efficiently, which allows them to exercise at a higher intensity for longer periods of time.

To improve VO2 max, engage in regular aerobic exercise such as running, swimming, or cycling. Gradually increase the intensity and duration of your workouts over time. Consider incorporating interval training sessions, which alternate between high-intensity bursts and recovery periods.

Measure VO2:

This test is performed in the laboratory where you wear a mask that measures the amount of oxygen you inhale and carbon dioxide you exhale while exercising on a treadmill or stationary bike at progressively increasing intensity until you reach exhaustion.

By monitoring the gaseous concentration, you can find out how many calories you burn at different levels of intensity. Your heart rate also gets measured.

By calculating the maximum heart rate (multiplying your age by 0.7 and then subtracting it from 220) and your oxygen consumption, these measurements help doctors to prescribe you the right form of exercise.

Exercise prescription is written using these mnemonics:

F: Frequency: How often

I: Intensity: Low, moderate, or high

T: Time: specific time of the day and duration of exercise

T: Type: Cardio/aerobic /anaerobic

E: Enjoyment: something you really enjoy

Think FITTE to stay fit when setting a goal for exercise.

Obesity Medical Association recommends at least 150 minutes of workout every week, which is an average of 30 minutes daily, at least 5 days a week, that could be at a stretch or 3 bouts of 10 minutes each, whatever works better for your schedule. Also recommended is 2 days of core strengthening and resistance exercises.

5.6 Workout That Works for Me

It is essential to start with a workout that you genuinely enjoy and that fits seamlessly into your schedule. For me, that could mean engaging in a lively dance class, where the rhythm and movement lift my spirits. Alternatively, I might opt for a calming yoga session to enhance my flexibility and mindfulness. On days when the weather is fine, I find joy in walking through my neighborhood or a local park, soaking in the fresh air and scenery.

Another option we love is hot yoga, where the warmth of the room allows for deeper stretches and relaxation. No matter the choice, the key is to select activities that resonate with you, making workouts not just a chore but a fulfilling part of your day. Finding an exercise you enjoy doing is the key to consistency. It helps you stay committed to your fitness journey.

ABC Technique:

A - Awareness → B - Behavior → C - Change

A - Awareness: From Sitting to Shifting

"Sitting is the new smoking - but awareness is the first rep."

This helps you recognize how inactivity affects health and understand why movement matters beyond weight loss.

Sedentary lifestyles, such as prolonged sitting, can significantly increase the risk for heart disease, obesity, diabetes, and depression - a phenomenon sometimes called "active couch potato syndrome," where one meets exercise guidelines but still spends too much time sitting overall. Engaging in regular exercise is important not only because it improves metabolism, insulin sensitivity, mood, energy, sleep, and longevity, but also because it protects the brain, strengthens bones, and boosts confidence. Ultimately, the most powerful transformation comes from shifting our mindset about movement: instead of seeing it as a punishment ("I have to exercise"), embracing it as an opportunity ("I get to move") empowers us to make activity a meaningful and joyful part of everyday life.

Reflections:

- How much time do I spend sitting each day - and how does it affect how I feel?

____

____

____

____

____

- What's one way movement has helped my physical or mental health in the past?

____

____

____

____

____

- What has kept me from starting or staying consistent?

____

____

____

____

____

B - Behavior: Just Get Moving

"The best workout is the one you'll do - consistently."

Now it is time to go from thinking about movement to taking manageable, personalized action.

When it comes to getting started with movement, the key is not to overthink it - simply walk for five minutes, stretch, or dance in your kitchen. Focus on consistency rather than intensity: begin where you are and use whatever resources you have on hand. For those seeking structure, short, seven-minute full-body routines are great for beginners and can be done at home using just bodyweight, resistance bands, or free online resources like YouTube workouts. Incorporate both cardio activities - such as brisk walking, cycling, or swimming - to get your heart rate up, and core exercises like planks, bridges, or pelvic stability work to build a foundation for posture and back health. Common barriers include feeling short on time, fatigue, or a dislike of the gym, but these can often be overcome with at-home options, enjoyable activities, or breaking movement into smaller, manageable segments.

Reflections:

- What's one small form of movement I enjoy or could try today?

- How can I fit 10 minutes of activity into my current schedule?

____

____

____

____

____

- How does movement make me feel emotionally?

____

____

____

____

____

C - Change: Building an Active Identity

"You don't need to lift heavy - just stay light on your feet."

In this stage, movement becomes part of who you are, not just something you do.

Finding a workout that works for you can be as simple as exploring walking, dancing, yoga, biking, strength training, or Pilates - choose what fits your lifestyle and mood. Consider creating a personal movement menu with options tailored for times when you're tired, busy, or feeling energized. Adopting an identity-based approach, such as seeing yourself as someone who moves daily rather than someone who "should exercise more," can help solidify lasting habits. Integrate activity into your existing routines - for example, pair a walk with a favorite podcast or do squats while your coffee brews. Most importantly, celebrate every micro-win along the way: a five-minute stretch or a habit streak are both achievements worth recognizing.

Reflections:

- What kind of movement makes me feel like me?

____

____

____

____

____

- What are my top 3 "go-to" activities when time or energy is limited?

____

____

____

____

____

- How will I celebrate consistency, not perfection?

Chapter : 6

Medications and Surgery

"It is part of the cure to wish to be cured."

-Seneca

TOOLS, NOT SHORTCUTS

In our experience, for many people, lifestyle changes such as improved nutrition, physical activity, and behavior modification are enough to bring about meaningful transformation. But sometimes, no matter how hard we try - changing how we eat, moving more, breaking old habits - the weight just doesn't come off. Or it does, only to creep back again. This is not a sign of weakness or failure. It is just a reflection of the complex biology of obesity: metabolism, hormones, inflammation, and genetics all play a powerful role.

In such cases, there are additional tools - **weight-loss medications and bariatric surgery** - to help bridge the gap between your effort and outcome. These tools aren't quick fixes or shortcuts. They are evidence-based ways to help your body work with you in your journey toward better health.

Medications can help calm cravings, control appetite, and rebalance the signals that drive weight gain. Surgery can do even more - it changes not only the size of the stomach but also the hormones that affect hunger, metabolism, and blood sugar. Both approaches can be lifesaving when applied thoughtfully, in the right context, and with the right support.

But here's the key: medications and surgery are not the

whole journey. They are powerful tools that work best when combined with the habits and mindset shifts, we've been talking about throughout this book. Think of them as opening the door. You still need to walk through, but now the path is clearer and the steps lighter.

6.1 Weight loss Medications

Why medications?

Medications play a significant role in weight management, especially when it is challenging to make changes on our own. By incorporating medication into our weight loss journey, we are not solely relying on willpower. Certain medications can help regulate hormones that influence appetite and cravings.

Many patients using medications report that their preoccupation with food diminishes significantly. These medications help reduce cravings and enable individuals to focus on developing healthier habits, making it easier to manage their eating patterns.

These medications work on the hunger center of the brain, located deep inside a region called the hypothalamus, which sits near the base of the brain just above the neck. The hypothalamus regulates hunger, fullness, and energy balance.

Appetite control works like a gas pedal and a brake:

- POMC/CART pathway *(Pro-opiomelanocortin / Cocaine- and Amphetamine-Regulated Transcript)* is the **brake.** When activated, it increases feelings of fullness and reduces appetite.

- AgRP/NPY pathway *(Agouti-Related Peptide / Neuropeptide Y)* is the **accelerator.** When active, it increases hunger and food-seeking behavior.

Weight-loss medications help restore balance by slowing the accelerator, pressing the brakes, or both, making hunger easier to control , reduce cravings, and make lifestyle changes easier to maintain.

Please remember that the focus of this book is not to direct you to any specific prescription medications. This is just to give you an idea about the various medications available in the market. Do consult your physician for any weight loss medications.

Medications are taking the front seat in weight management. With the invention **of GLP-1 (Glucagon-Like Peptides), a medication that helps with weight loss by reducing appetite and decreasing gut motility hence there is a huge demand for this medication all over the United States and other countries.** In recent years, GLP-1s have surged in popularity - more than 286,000 prescriptions were written in 2023 alone, with demand climbing even higher in 2024–2025. But high costs, limited insurance coverage, and availability issues have left many people without access to these.

You can always talk to your provider. If you are taking any medications, discuss their potential side effects. Observe the precautions that have to be taken while consuming these medications. We will start with the most popular ones.

How does it work?

GLP/GIP: (Glucagon-Like Peptide-1 and Glucose-Dependent Insulinotropic Polypeptide)

This medication works on the gut, reducing the mobility and also stimulating your pancreas to release more insulin, which helps in diabetes. When food is staying longer in the gut, the gut is constantly talking to the brain, and gives you a feeling of being full for longer hours.

Also, it works on the hunger center in the brain to decrease appetite. Both of these mechanisms make this class effective in controlling appetite. I keep hearing from my patients taking these medications that their food cravings have decreased.

The patient taking this medication will feel full for longer periods. The appetite slows down. I have to make them more aware of their protein intake. While taking this medication, you have to be careful about some side effects, including but not limited to nausea, constipation, vomiting, and abdominal pain.

At the time of writing, these medications carry a black box warning about a potential risk of thyroid cancer. It's important to discuss this carefully with your healthcare provider before starting treatment.

Coverage for this medication is the biggest limiting factor. Talk to your provider if you could be an appropriate candidate for this medication. It is a good idea to check with your insurance company for its coverage before even making an appointment with your physician.

Another commonly used medication in this class is phentermine. You may remember 'Phen-Fen,' a drug combination popular in the 1970s that was later banned because of side effects linked to the fenfluramine component - not phentermine itself. Phentermine is still available today, but because it is a controlled substance, it should only be used under close medical supervision and regular monitoring by your physician.

Another class of medication is a combination of Wellbutrin and naltrexone. It works really well for issues related to emotional eating. This medication is not considered for patients with h/o seizure disorder.

Medications have the benefits of cutting down the appetite, but also some side effects that you should be aware of. Please have a detailed discussion with the prescribing provider before starting.

Orlistat

Orlistat works by decreasing fat absorption from the diet, inhibiting a hormone called lipase. It causes flatulence and foul-smelling stools condition called steatorrhea. It is better to watch fat intake while taking this medication.

Medications are an adjunct to lifestyle interventions. I always use it as an additional tool while working with the patient on diet and physical activity. Medications are certainly helpful. However, actively working on behavioral aspects and eating habits is crucial in this journey.

6.2 Bariatric Surgery

Weight loss surgeries are becoming more and more common with time. Due to advancements in procedures and technology, we see more awareness regarding weight management. The effective results of bariatric surgery make it the most popular.

Weight loss surgeries are usually taken as a measure when people fail at conservative measures. The American Society of Bariatric Surgery and Metabolic Diseases (ASMBS) has set some guidelines for candidates who are deemed eligible to undergo this surgery. They are as follows:

- Anyone having a BMI above 35
- Anyone with a BMI above 30 with metabolic disease

While bariatric surgery could indeed be helpful, it also needs some prior preparation, discipline, and work-up before insurance companies can cover it. Usually, you need to get established with a bariatric surgeon and get enrolled in the medical weight management or try that for 3 to 6 months before surgery could be performed.

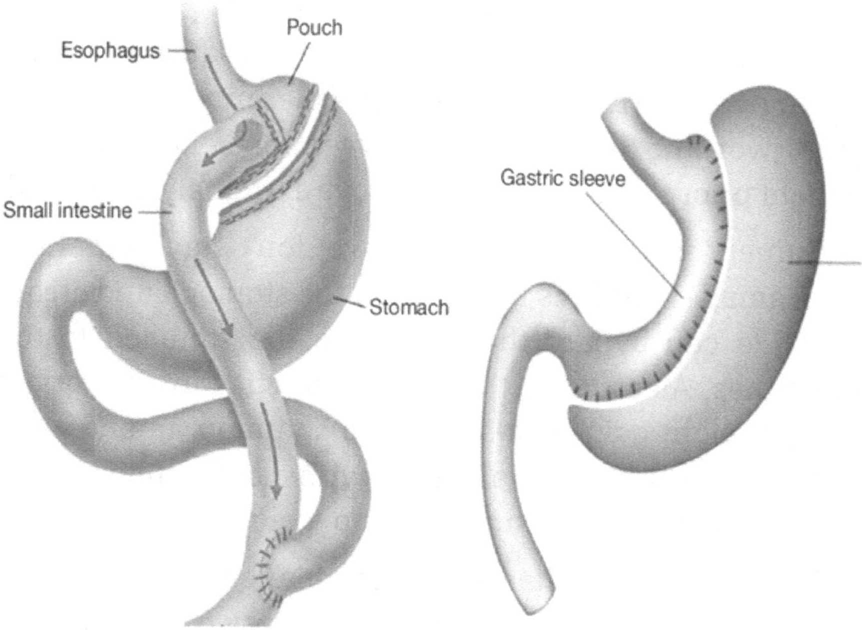

In sleeve gastrectomy, a part of the stomach is removed, and a small pouch of 50 cc is created that limits food intake.

Another useful surgery is called Roux-en-Y, in which a part of the stomach is cut to create a pouch. That part is bypassed to the third part of intestine.

Before performing bariatric surgery, you would need to have an evaluation from a psychiatrist. You need to understand complete diet education, sleep evaluation, and possibly need an EGD. You would also need to get established with a nutritionist.

Once surgery is performed, it is important to stay compliant with dietary changes. This entails eating smaller portions and frequent small meals. It is also important to take vitamins, as certain parts of the intestines help in absorbing multivitamins during bypass. If you had a bariatric surgery or are planning to have one, start working on lifestyle interventions. Losing some weight prior to the surgery can prove extremely beneficial.

Surgery is not a quick fix. If we don't stay compliant with smaller portions in diet, then the stomach and create a fistula can bypass the food from the stomach to the intestines. As a result, the restrictive effect of surgery is gone. Weight gain post-surgery is common among such cases. Thus, timely evaluation with your primary care physician or bariatric surgeon for a weight check is vital.

Take your multivitamins, additional calcium, vitamin D, and iron. Checking vitamin levels every 6 months with the PCP is important.

If despite having a bariatric surgery, you are still regaining lost weight or experiencing any abdominal pain, this could be a sign of dumping syndrome. This can happen if you eat too fast and experience post-bariatric surgery hypoglycemia. The reason for regaining weight could be the development of a fistula between the stomach and the intestine. There are no restrictive effects of bariatric surgery. If you eat as much as you wish, it would obviously lead to weight regain.

If you are experiencing these symptoms, please talk to your provider. Certain conditions need to be ruled out. Blood work can be performed to discover any vitamin deficiencies. Eating smaller portions of meals, slow eating, complex carbohydrates, and decreasing sugar intake are key points that can really help you sustain weight loss after surgery.

Over the course of past several years, we have witnessed the struggles and successes of many patients. We have seen patients not only lose weight but also get better overall, having successfully countered obesity related health conditions. With its ability to instill discipline and change bad dietary habits, bariatric surgery could be absolutely life-changing, meaning a new lease of life.

GLP medications and semaglutides can also prove to be helpful in controlling weight after weight loss surgery.

ABC Technique:

A - Awareness → B - Behavior → C - Change

A - Awareness: Medical Tools for a Medical Condition

"Obesity is a chronic and medically treatable condition, not a character flaw."

This helps you understand the science and role of medications and surgery in obesity treatment.

When lifestyle changes alone aren't enough, it's important to recognize that genetics, biology, hormones, and set point theory all play significant roles, making obesity a chronic, relapsing condition that often requires long-term care. Medical weight loss tools, such as FDA-approved anti-obesity medications—including GLP-1 receptor agonists like semaglutide and tirzepatide - work by regulating appetite, improving insulin sensitivity, and signaling satiety. These medications are generally considered for individuals with a BMI of 30 or higher, or 27 and above if other medical conditions are present. Bariatric surgery, an option for those with a BMI of 40 or greater, or 35 with obesity-related conditions like diabetes or sleep apnea, includes procedures such as sleeve gastrectomy, gastric bypass, and duodenal switch, all of which rely on hormonal changes to reduce hunger and improve metabolic health. It's essential to challenge stigma and misconceptions around these interventions; choosing medication or surgery is not a sign of weakness, but rather an empowered step toward taking control of your health with the right tools.

Reflections:

- Have I ever judged myself or others for using medical weight loss tools?

____

____

____

____

____

- What's holding me back from considering medication or surgery as valid options?

____

____

____

____

- What would it mean to ask for help, medically or surgically?

____

____

____

____

____

B - Behavior: Making an Informed, Empowered Decision

"The right choice is the one that aligns with your goals, health, and values."

This stage helps you gather the facts, talk to their care team, and integrate treatments with behavioral support.

When exploring your options with your doctor, it's important to know which questions to ask about medications or surgery so you can fully understand the risks, benefits, and expectations involved. For those considering medication support, daily or weekly dosing routines—such as proper injection techniques—become part of your new health regimen, alongside learning to manage potential side effects like nausea, constipation, or fatigue. Integrating these medications effectively means pairing them with mindful eating, self-tracking, and regular movement. If you are preparing for surgery, it's crucial to understand how your lifestyle will change post-surgery, from adjusting your eating pace and portion sizes to incorporating necessary supplements. After treatment, continuing supportive behaviors like journaling, meal planning, therapy, and participating in support groups will be key. Ongoing self-monitoring for emotional eating patterns or shifts such as "addiction transfer" will support your long-term success.

Reflections:

- What are my biggest hopes and fears about weight loss medication or surgery?

____

____

____

____

____

- How ready am I to follow the behavioral guidelines that support these treatments?

____

____

____

____

____

- How do I want to feel – not just physically, but emotionally – one year from now?

____

____

____

____

____

C - Change: Living Lighter with Medical Support

"Medications and surgery are tools - not magic. But with commitment, they change lives."

This helps you understand long-term transformation, identity shifts, and post-treatment success - including emotional and lifestyle support.

Sustaining change after medications or surgery requires more than a reset of biology - lasting progress comes from the habits you build and maintain. Preventing weight regain involves ongoing coaching, regular check-ins, and the support of cognitive behavioral therapy (CBT) to reinforce healthy routines. Addressing the emotional layers of this journey is also essential, as weight loss often leads to questions of identity - "Who am I now that I've lost weight?" - and can bring shifts in attention, family dynamics, and body image. Therapy may be helpful in working through feelings of grief, trauma, or self-worth. As you move forward, it becomes important to redefine success beyond the number on the scale, celebrating improvements in energy, mobility, confidence, health, and the non-scale victories such as how your clothes fit, lab results, strength, and a sense of freedom. Long-term support may come from registered dietitians, support groups, bariatric coaches, and accountability partners, all working with you to ensure your continued growth and maintenance of positive changes.

Reflections:

- How will I measure success beyond the number on the scale?

____

____

____

____

____

- How can I honor the hard work I've done - with or without surgery/medication?

____

____

____

____

____

- What does "living lighter" mean to me now?

Chapter : 7

Weight Loss Plateau

"Success is not final, failure is not fatal: it is the courage to continue that counts."

- Winston Churchill

THE PAUSE BEFORE THE NEXT SHIFT

Weight loss plateaus are a common experience, where progress comes to a standstill in spite of continued efforts.

We have observed this often in my patients. After losing a significant amount of weight or even after losing a few pounds, the weight scale simply refuses to budge. People find this to be extremely frustrating.

Let us understand why we hit a weight plateau.

1. As we lose more weight, our metabolism sometimes goes down, especially if we are not doing any metabolism-enhancing exercises.
2. When we cut down all carbohydrates, our body has a natural tendency to conserve more energy.
3. Another reason for weight plateau is that our body tends to slow down the motility of the gut constipation. This is common in the weight loss journey.
4. Our body tends to preserve maximum calories.

How to break a weight plateau?

Depending upon the BMI, sometimes I ask patients to focus on a healthy diet, keeping up with protein and healthy carbohydrate intake, and keeping up with physical activity goals instead of really focusing on the numbers.

To overcome a weight plateau, try the following strategies:

Diet:

- Maintain a moderate calorie-deficient diet
- Increase protein intake
- Add fiber to your meals
- Limit processed foods and sugary drinks

Exercise:

- Aim for 150 minutes of moderate or 75 minutes of vigorous activity each week
- Try new exercises like HIIT, strength training, or dance

Medications:

- Discuss with your healthcare provider about medications

Address Psychological Factors:

- Stress
- Relaxation and medication techniques
- Hire a coach
- Celebrate your success

Here is a list of foods that can enhance our metabolism and help break the weight plateau.

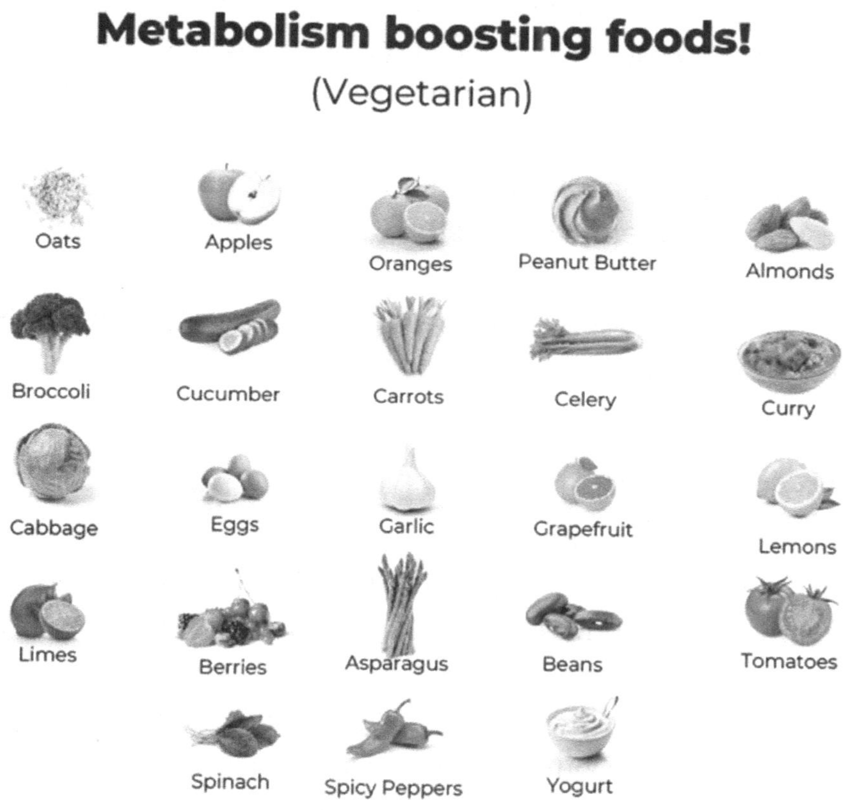
Metabolism boosting foods!
(Vegetarian)
Oats
Apples
Oranges
Peanut Butter
Almonds
Broccoli
Cucumber
Carrots
Celery
Curry
Cabbage
Eggs
Garlic
Grapefruit
Lemons
Limes
Berries
Asparagus
Beans
Tomatoes
Spinach
Spicy Peppers
Yogurt

Here are some additional diets to keep in consideration that help in losing weight.

7.1 Intermittent Fasting

Most diets focus on what you eat. Intermittent fasting focuses on when you eat. With intermittent fasting, you only eat during a specific time. There is enough data showing that fasting for a certain number of hours each day or eating just one meal in a couple of days a week may have health benefits.

In prehistoric times, hunters were forced to remain hungry for long periods of time. They evolved to survive and thrive for longer periods without eating. They had to work hard to hunt and find food. Even now, before the introduction of computers and phones, we did not have this epidemic of obesity. It all started with the easy availability of food, 24/7 entertainment, the introduction of sweet beverages, staying awake for longer night hours, frequent snacking, and eating all day.

How does it work?

During fasting hours, the body can start using fats as an energy source. Johns Hopkins neuroscientist, Mark Mattson, has studied intermittent fasting for over 25 years. He says our bodies have evolved to be able to survive for hours together without food. The body exhausts its sugar stores and starts burning fat. He refers to this as metabolic switching. The body starts burning fat once it has exhausted the calories consumed during the last meal.

Intermittent fasting contrasts with the normal eating pattern for most Americans, who eat throughout their waking hours. Mattson says, "If someone is eating three meals a day, plus snacks, and they are not exercising, then every time they eat, they are running on those calories and not burning their fat store.

Popular Ways to do Intermittent Fasting

- **Time Restricted** 16:8: In this, you can eat within a window of 8 hours and fast for the next 16 hours.
- **Alternate day fasting.**
- **5:2 approach:** This involves eating regularly five days a week. For the other two days, you limit yourself to one 500-600 calorie meal. An example would be if you chose to eat normally on every day of the week except Mondays and Thursdays, which would be your one-meal days.
- **Eat, stop, eat.**
- **Warrior diet:** This diet is a type of intermittent fasting that shows bursts of overeating after long periods of under-eating. This pattern is inappropriate for many people and may lead to disordered eating. This is not supported by many studies. I do not advise this pattern of eating.
- **Spontaneously skipping meals.**

The most important question in intermittent fasting is what to eat and what not to eat during the fasting time. During fasting periods, you may have water, black coffee or tea.

During the eating hours, nutrition experts suggest a Mediterranean-style diet. You cannot go wrong when you pick leafy greens, lean meats, whole grains, complex carbs, colored fruits and veggies, olive oils, healthy fats, quinoa, etc. If you are not mindful during eating time and keep filling yourself with high-calorie' junk food, you will not be able to lose weight.

Intermittent Fasting Benefits:

Intermittent fasting is more than just burning fat. It affects the body and brain as well.

It not only helps lose weight, but it also decreases insulin levels. It helps in reducing insulin resistance during fasting hours. The body uses stored fat and sugar as an energy source that helps in losing weight. When done properly, intermittent fasting can help improve metabolic health and reduce the risk of conditions such as type 2 diabetes, coronary heart disease, inflammatory bowel disease, and fatty liver disease.

Most of the available research shows that intermittent fasting can help people lose body weight and lower their levels of fasting glucose and leptin. It decreases insulin resistance and drops levels of leptin while simultaneously increasing levels of adiponectin. It can help in reducing insulin needs.

It can take two to four weeks before the body gets accustomed to intermittent fasting. You might feel hungry or cranky while you are getting used to the new routine. The people who stick to the plan and remain persistent feel better at the end.

It is observed in many cultures, that fasting one day a week is quite common. Though it is a new concept for Western countries, but benefits of 1 day a week fasting have been mentioned and routinely practiced in many cultures.

7.2 Think before you drink!

Mr. James walked into his first appointment looking nervous. He greeted with a big smile. It had been a while since he had seen a doctor. As a retired single man, he had lived life on his own terms. However, when we looked at his lab results, we were taken aback to see that his A1c was 10.2. He didn't realize he had diabetes and hadn't visited a doctor for over a decade or so.

During our chat about his diet, he revealed that he was drinking 6 cans of a sweet sugary soda every day! When we asked him to confirm that, his immediate reaction was, "Don't ask me to stop drinking my favorite soda. This is the only fun I have in my life!" So, we came up with a friendly deal. He would drink a glass of water before having the soda. We also started him on some diabetic medications, and we made that one commitment about water.

We were thrilled to see that within just three months; he managed to lower his A1c from 10.2 to 6.2 and was almost ready to give up on his favorite soda. It was a simple trick that worked wonders. We personally liked it so much that we started using it with other patients, and most of them were happy to give it a try instead of just being told to quit their favorite sodas.

This is one example, but we see lots of patients with high A1c and weight issues. Invariably, they too are in the habit of drinking too many sweet sugary beverages (SSBs). The main issue with liquid sweeteners is that it is easily absorbed and ready to be used as an energy source. If not, then they get stored in the form of fat.

Around 60% of our body consists of water. What is in the glass that we hold matters a lot. The two most commonly consumed types of drinks in the USA are sweet sugary beverages (SSBs) and juices. We will dig deeper in the content and ingredients of such beverages.

According to the US Framingham Heart Study (2020), regular SSB intake was associated with adverse changes in cholesterol. It can further increase cardiovascular risks. Here is the reference for this study.

1 Can = 270 calories = 1 pound in 13 days = 28 pounds a year

Let us go over the individual contents of your favorite soda can:

Sugar: 39 g, average 10 teaspoons, causes a spike in insulin level. Extra sugar causes fat production in the body. One teaspoon of sugar contains 15 calories, so 10 teaspoons would contain 150 calories.

Phosphoric acid: Erodes tooth enamel.

Caffeine: Works as a diuretic and makes you dehydrated.

Aspartame: Artificial sweetener. Highly acidic.

What happens after you drink a can of regular soda?

- Sugar spikes within 10 minutes, and then the insulin level starts rising.
- After 20 minutes of the sugar spike, he did not

immediately vomit because of the phosphoric acid content. Your insulin level spikes. The liver responds to that by turning any extra sugar into fat.

- In the next 40 to 45 minutes, caffeine absorption causes the pupils to dilate and raises blood pressure. Dopamine production also increases during this time. This is the stimulating pleasure center of the brain, which gives a feeling of euphoria.
- In the following 60 minutes, phosphoric acid binds to calcium. Magnesium and zinc make it unavailable for bone growth. Calcium and phosphorus bind together and get deposited in the kidneys, causing stones.
- After 1 hour, caffeine's diuretic property makes you urinate more and dehydrates your body.

So, a can of soda is not hydrating you at all. Actually, it is making you more dehydrated. I see that in my practice, a lot of people drink soda instead of water, thinking that it is hydrating the body, whereas it actually does the exact opposite.

Americans consume 22 teaspoons of added sugar every day. That is nearly 400% of the daily recommended amount.

Most commonly available sweet soft drinks contain anywhere between 25 to 60 grams of sugar!

Healthy Alternatives:

- Kombucha: Have you ever heard of this? Look it up!
- Iced tea or hot tea
- Sparkling water
- Sparkling lemonade
- Freshly squeezed lemonade
- Maple water
- Water infusions with fruit and herbs for flavor
- Mineral water
- Coconut water

For example, most of us are picky about our clothes. Why are we so liberal in making a decision of what goes inside our body? Say it like you mean it! My body contains 60% of liquids. I am going to choose my drink wisely.

It is extremely important to pay attention to the liquid in our bodies. It is needed not only for hydration, but also for lubrication of our joints, muscle hydration, cleansing the kidneys, metabolism, and multiple other functions.

Carbonated drinks are commonly seen as popular drinking beverages. Let us take a look at the contents. They believe they can have it as much as possible.

Here are some of the ingredients in your favorite soda can

- **Phosphoric acid:** Calcium and phosphoric acid affect the kidneys. Calcium phosphate causes kidney stones.
- **Yellow dye:** Could be a health concern in children as

well as adults.

- **Aspartame:** This can be associated with bladder cancer.

Similarly, as noted above, most of the carbonated drinks contain a lot of sugar. Artificial sweeteners make it even worse.

pH of the liquid

We get a lot of questions about alkaline water. Alkaline water has a higher pH (usually 8-9) compared to regular drinking water (pH ~7). It's marketed as being able to neutralize acid in the body, improve metabolism, increase energy, and even help with weight loss.

What we know:

- **Hydration matters most:** Drinking adequate water is essential for metabolism, digestion, and appetite control. Some studies suggest water (alkaline or not) before meals may promote satiety and reduce calorie intake.
- **Alkalinity claims are unproven:** The body tightly regulates blood pH through the lungs and kidneys. There is no strong evidence that alkaline water significantly changes body pH or improves fat burning.
- **Limited research:** A few small studies suggest possible antioxidant effects and slight improvements in blood sugar or cholesterol markers, but results are

inconsistent and not robust enough to confirm benefits for weight loss.

- **Safety:** Generally safe in moderation, but excessive intake could alter mineral balance, particularly in people with kidney issues.

How much water should I drink?

On average, we need 60 ounces of water every day. This is a highlighted point in our practice. Drinking water is good for hydration. Oftentimes, we are more thirsty than hungry. The brain receives the signal. Instead of drinking water, you eat something. This causes weight gain. So, the next time you feel hungry, have a glass of water instead. After a while, if you still feel hungry, you can have something light.

7.3 Meal Replacements:

Meal Replacements (MRs)

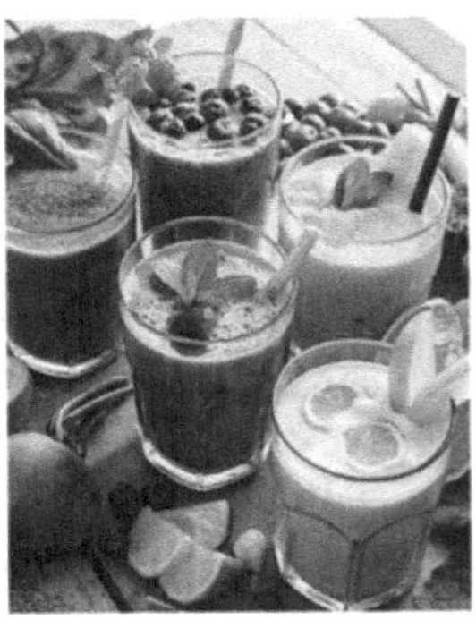

- Prepackaged Food Product
- Portion-Controlled
- High Nutrition
- Calories-Controlled

Clinical MRs typically have:

- Protein- 215 g
- Fiber- 25 g
- Sugar- < 7g

A meal replacement is a pre-packaged food product, such as a shake, bar, or soup, that typically contains a controlled portion of calories and essential nutrients. These products are designed to provide a balanced diet without the need for extensive meal preparation. Meal replacements are often used in lifestyle interventions for weight management and can substitute for a regular meal. They are an effective way to ensure adequate nutrition and can aid in weight loss, particularly in a culture where high-carbohydrate and high-fat foods are easily accessible. People often have busy lifestyles with little time to cook.

Pros of Meal Replacement Shakes

Full of nutrients: Due to being portion-controlled and fixed calories and nutrients, one way to get enough nutrition in terms of proteins, carbohydrates, and fiber.

Low calories: Most MRs are controlled on the calories (lower side), so they can help obtain enough protein. A meal replacement shake is a good addition to your diet if you are watching your weight or trying to lose weight. As they are rich in proteins, they help in overcoming the obstacle of feeling hungry while on a low-calorie diet.

Handy: MRs are easy to prepare and consume. They could be handy, especially in a busy work culture.

Added fiber: In addition to protein, which helps you feel full, meal replacement shakes are often high in fiber. This helps healthy digestion, so that you don't feel bloated or have constipation.

There is enough research proving that using meal replacement could help in losing weight. Here are some cons.

Cons of Meal Replacement Shakes

Meal replacement shakes often contain artificial ingredients to enhance flavor and preserve nutrients, along with added sugars for taste. Thus, it is important to check labels for quality. Aim for at least 3 grams of fiber and a higher protein content than carbohydrates. While these shakes typically range from 150 to 200 calories, which can aid in weight loss, it is important to ensure that you are still getting enough calories from other meals and snacks. They are high in protein, which helps you to feel satisfied without consuming excessive calories.

Meal replacements can be effective for weight loss when combined with a lifestyle change. They can help you feel full while eating fewer calories.

7.4 Glycemic Index

The glycemic index (GI) is a scale that ranks carbohydrate foods based on how quickly they raise blood sugar levels. There is a number assigned from 0-100, with pure glucose having a GI of 100. It's a tool to help people manage their blood sugar, especially those with diabetes or pre-diabetes.

Low GI (0-55): These foods cause a slower and smaller

rise in blood sugar. It includes most fruits and vegetables, beans, minimally processed grains, pasta, low-fat dairy, and nuts.

Medium GI (56-69): These foods cause a moderate rise in blood sugar, such as white and sweet potatoes, corn, white rice, couscous, and some breakfast cereals.

High GI (70 or higher): These foods cause a rapid and significant rise in blood sugar, including white bread, rice cakes, most crackers, bagels, cakes, doughnuts, croissants, and most packaged breakfast cereals.

Switching to foods with low GI can help in weight loss as well as weight maintenance. Please refer to the chart to find the GI for a particular food.

It's important to note that the GI doesn't account for the amount of carbohydrate in a serving, which is where glycemic load (GL) comes into play. GL considers both the GI and the amount of carbohydrate in a serving. Refer to the picture below for a list of foods based on their glycemic index.

Remember weight loss plateau can take time to break, and it needs patience and persistence. Intermittent fasting, low glycemic index foods, more intense workouts, watching your sugar and sweet beverages, or even adding or changing weight loss medications could be a help in achieving better health.

ABC Technique: Breaking Through a Weight Loss Plateau

A - Awareness → B - Behavior → C - Change

A - Awareness: Why Plateaus Happen

"A plateau is not failure - it's feedback."

Please understand that plateaus are normal, physiological, and adjustable, not a sign you're your efforts have failed.

As you work to break through a weight loss plateau, it's helpful to understand why the body plateaus in the first place. Factors like adaptive thermogenesis - where your body becomes more efficient at a lower weight - as well as muscle loss, decreased non-exercise activity, and general metabolic slowdown all contribute. The mindset trap is another hurdle; frustration can easily spiral into all-or-nothing thinking, binge cycles, or even giving up altogether. Paying attention to your glycemic index (GI) is also crucial. Not all carbohydrates are created equal - GI impacts blood sugar, hunger, and fat storage, so opting for lower-GI foods such as lentils, oats, or berries can help you feel fuller longer and reduce insulin spikes, supporting your progress on this journey.

Reflections:

- How does it feel when the scale doesn't move – and what story do I tell myself?

- Am I tracking things beyond the scale – energy, strength, consistency?

- What's one area I've stopped paying attention to since I started this journey?

B - Behavior: Fine-Tuning for Progress

"Small, smart adjustments beat extreme overhauls."

Identify realistic behavioral tweaks that can reignite your progress without restriction or burnout.

When navigating a weight loss plateau, there are several effective adjustments you can consider. Intermittent fasting - using methods like 16:8, 14:10, or 5:2 - can support insulin sensitivity and help regulate appetite by encouraging mindful eating within set windows, rather than promoting restriction. Paying close attention to beverage choices is important too, as sugary drinks, sweetened teas, juices, and alcohol contribute hidden calories that rarely provide satiety and can easily be overconsumed. For those with busy schedules or a desire for greater portion control, meal replacements such as high-protein, low-GI shakes or fiber-rich bars can be practical options. Reassessing your carbohydrate quality is also beneficial: opting for lower-GI choices like quinoa in place of white rice or berries instead of juice, and pairing carbohydrates with protein or healthy fats, helps stabilize blood sugar and prolongs fullness. These mindful, sustainable changes can help reignite progress and reinforce your healthy habits.

Reflections:

- Have I been drinking calories without noticing?

- Would trying a meal replacement help simplify my food choices – or feel too restrictive?

- How could I gently experiment with intermittent fasting?

C - Change: Staying the Course with Strategy & Patience

"There are no roadblocks - only turning points to refine, reset, and rise higher."

Now rebuilds momentum through sustainable upgrades, mindset reinforcement, and celebrating progress beyond the scale.

Tracking progress beyond the scale is essential - non-scale victories like improved lab results, clothes fitting better, enhanced sleep quality, and greater mental clarity are all signs of forward momentum. When making changes, prioritize strategic, modest upgrades over drastic measures. For example, consider closing the kitchen at 8 PM or swapping your nightly glass of wine for herbal tea a few nights a week. Remember that personalization is key, as not every tool will work for everyone - embrace a spirit of experimentation, observe what works, and make adjustments accordingly. Above all, recognize that staying consistent, rather than being perfect, is what keeps you in the game; plateaus often signal that a breakthrough is near.

Reflections:

- What progress have I made that isn't showing up on the scale?

- What's one small change I can commit to this week to move forward?

- What new identity am I building - and how would that version of me respond right now?

Final Reflections from the Authors

"As you start to walk on the way, the way appears."

-Rumi

In this book, we set out to share the foundational concepts of weight management and healthy living - practical steps that anyone can begin to apply in daily life to lose weight and improve overall health. Think of this book as a toolkit: one you can return to at any time, at your own pace, to guide and support your journey.

We began with the basics - understanding your own body and recognizing the impact of unhealthy weight gain on long-term health. From there, we explored how to make better choices with food, how to understand and reshape mindset and behavior, and how to build motivation that lasts. We emphasized exercise, often the hardest habit to establish, and walked through practical ways to make movement a natural part of your life. We also touched on medications - not as medical advice, but as one of the many tools available today - and acknowledged that, for some, weight loss surgery may serve as a fifth pillar alongside the four pillars of diet, exercise, behavior, and medication.

Our hope is that Living Lighter does more than provide knowledge. We hope it sparks awareness - awareness of your own health, of the role obesity plays as a disease in our society, and of the collective action we can take to build healthier lives for ourselves and our loved ones.

Remember, change doesn't happen all at once. It happens step by step - through awareness, through better choices, and through the courage to keep moving forward. If this book has given you even one insight, one shift in mindset, or one tool you can use on your journey, then it has served its purpose.

We invite you to take what you've learned, apply it with compassion for yourself, and share it with others. Together, we can begin to change the narrative around weight, health, and well-being - one lighter step at a time.

As you go through this journey, please remember!

You are a beautiful and blissful being by nature. Weight is just a number for the gravitational force working on your body. Let's ensure that we continue being kind and compassionate to ourselves and everyone around us.

With Love and gratitude!

Kavita & Sandeep